Medicine in the American Colonies

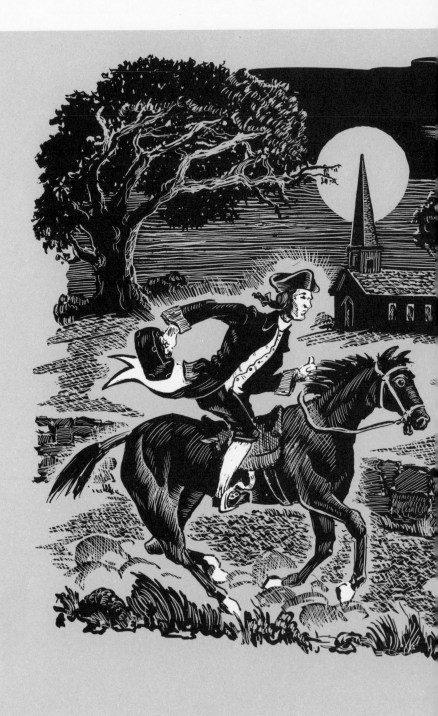

MEDICINE IN THE AMERICAN COLONIES

An
Historical Sketch of the
State of Medicine in the
American Colonies, From
Their First Settlement to
the Period of the
Revolution
By

DR. JOHN B. BECK

Foreword By

DR. CHARLES F. FISHBACK
OF LOVELACE CLINIC

Original Printed in Albany, New York, 1850

HORN & WALLACE
Publishers

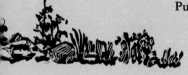

Horn & Wallace Publishers, Inc.
P.O. Box 4204, Albuquerque, New Mexico

CONTENTS

FOREWORD

THE ALMOST UNBELIEVABLE STORY OF THE GROWTH OF medicine from the time of the first American settlement to the Revolutionary War could fill a number of books. The subject itself is a fascinating one—the story of the astonishing progress that was made in such a few brief years, in the face of tremendous prejudice and ignorance at every hand; but more than that, Dr. John Broadhead Beck's book is thoroughly comprehensive and "alive" even after the passage of so many years.

Originally the material in this volume was presented by Dr. Beck before the New York State Medical Society in 1850. The development of medicine in those early years seems almost an impossibility, considering the problems facing it. The daring experiments carried out by the doctors of that time were often made upon a physician's own family, and they equal in courage the exploits of other fearless Colonists.

Dr. Beck was fully qualified in his day as one of the leaders in the field of medicine. He was professor of medicine at the College of Physicians and Surgeons in New York, seventeenth President of the New York Medical Society (1841), and was best known as an historian of the early days of medicine. He was born September 18, 1794, and graduated in 1817 from the College of Physicians and Surgeons of New York where his thesis on "Infanticide" was subsequently incorporated into a great work on medical jurisprudence. In 1822 he established the New York Medical and Physical Journal, and in 1824 he became the pro-

fessor of Materia Medica and Botany in his College. There
he published a volume on "Infantile Therapeutics" in
1848. In his lectures he stressed that it was wiser to be
"judicious in the use of a few remedies, than able to over-
whelm disease by a multitude of them."

Early medicine in this country did not resemble in any
particular the modern concept in this field. Today, the use
of the word "medicine" conjures visions of doctors, hospitals, research, specialized practice and regulation. In the
early Colonies, however, the "medical profession was in a
low and degraded condition," involving neither lectures
nor hospitals. The earliest practitioners in the Colonies
were the clergy. By 1649 so many completely unqualified
men were preaching the healing arts that the Colony of
Massachusetts passed a law which was the first attempt to
"put a restraint upon those who pretended to the practice
of physic." Soon thereafter, the State of New York developed the first truly effective measure for the regulation of
the practice of medicine which included certification and
penalties. In 1772 New Jersey passed a similar law. These
were the only Colonies known to have established such
regulations.

The most remarkable event in those early years was the
introduction and practice of inoculation for smallpox. In
1721 this revolutionary new procedure was introduced by
a clergyman-doctor who tried it out on his own family. By
1738 vaccination was practiced generally in Charleston,
South Carolina, and statistical evaluation soon began. It
was estimated the deaths in New England from smallpox
prior to the institution of vaccination was approximately
one in 7 or 8 cases. After vaccination, the death rate drop-
ped to only one in 800 to 1000 cases.

With the growth of the scientific practice of medicine there soon began to appear medical publications. In 1677 Thomas Thatcher in Massachusetts published "A Brief Guide in the Small Pox and Measles." Benjamin Colman in 1721 also wrote on smallpox, and the first publication on pharmacy appeared in 1732. An excellent publication by Dr. William Douglass in 1736 on Scarlatina was of great medical value as late as 1850, while other medical subjects, such as tetanus, pathology, menses and gout were discussed in print. Since many of the early physicians had European educations, and access to European medical publications, their early writings were frequently published in foreign medical areas—Leyden, London and other cities. Eventually, however, articles on the subject appeared in this country, although there was no medical journal published here until after the War of Independence.

Prior to the Revolution there were only two hospitals in the Colonies and only the roughest rudiments of medical schools. Dr. Beck states that the "establishment of Medical Faculties was unquestionably the most important event which had yet taken place in the history of our Colonial Medicine." It was in 1752 that Philadelphia established a temporary hospital. The city of New York followed in 1769 by establishing a public hospital, due to the efforts of Dr. Samuel Bard. The trustees of Kings College in New York created a medical faculty in 1767 and granted the first medical degree, two years later. At the opening of Kings College medical school, Dr. Peter Middleton gave a practical lecture on croup.

In 1761 Dr. John Jones, known as the father of American Surgery, was given the first regular professorship of surgery in this country. He wisely presented ideas and ideals for qualifications required of a doctor. To quote: "A judicious surgeon will always find his powers and abilities of assisting the wretched proportionable to the time he has spent, and the pains he has bestowed in acquiring the proper knowledge of his profession." Dr. Jones is said to have been the personal physician of George Washington and Benjamin Franklin.

Thus we see the gradual beginning of modern medicine in America—superstition giving way to knowledge, scientific publications replacing emotional medical tracts, and centers for education, lectures and the collecting of medical data gaining respect from the average citizen. Medical growth in America continues to rank as one of the great miracles of this nation. The foresight and tremendous ability of a relative few, developed the groundwork, rules and ideals for present day physicians, giving us the background from which to carry the profession to even greater heights. Today this medical tradition is being carried forward by many, among the leaders being Dr. W. R. Lovelace and his nephew, the late Dr. W. R. Lovelace II. This spirit of ever pushing forward, onward is still essential to the life of the present day physician and the Art of Medicine.

Dr. Beck's book truly presents the reader with a glimpse of the basic, earliest roots of this spirit in America.

> Charles F. Fishback, B.S., B.M., M.S., M.D.
> Lovelace Clinic

Albuquerque, New Mexico
September, 1966

AN

HISTORICAL SKETCH

OF THE

STATE OF MEDICINE
IN THE AMERICAN COLONIES

From Their First Settlement to the
Period of the Revolution.

By

JOHN B. BECK, M. D.

Professor of Materia Medica and Medical Jurisprudence in the College of Physicians and Surgeons of the city of New York; Corresponding Member of the Royal Academy of Medicine of Paris; Corresponding Member of the Medical Society of London, etc., etc., etc.

SECOND EDITION

1850

NOTICE

THE substance of the following sketch was delivered a few years since, as the annual address before the State Medical Society. Since then, it has been revised and considerably enlarged. In its present form, it is hoped that it may not be an unacceptable offering to the profession, as a memorial of the early history of medicine in this country.

New York, February 1, 1850.

Chapter One

HISTORICAL SKETCH

THE PROFESSION OF MEDICINE MUST EVER OCCUPY A conspicuous station in the scientific history of a nation. Independently of its being devoted to purposes of high utility and exalted benevolence, the necessary alliance which there exists between medicine and the other departments of science, will always confer upon it a peculiar pre-eminence over every other professional pursuit. So intimate, indeed, has been this alliance, that we shall find on the one hand, medicine receiving laws in succession from philosophy, mathematics and chemistry; and on the other hand, the members of the medical profession will be recognized to have been, in every age and country, among the most successful cultivators of general science. What the effects of this association have been, it is not material at present to inquire. It is sufficient to state the fact itself, to show the importance of medical history. In this country, the history of medicine derives an additional interest from the striking illustration which it presents of the influence which our peculiar form of government exerts over the character and progress of science. It is unquestionably true, that our medicine participates largely of that spirit of independence, which characterizes the civil and political institutions of our country. It was not, however, until after the revolutionary war, that this was the case, when the medical mind of our country received an impulse to which it had

hitherto been a stranger. That portion of its history which
has been selected as the subject of the present sketch, was
not so fortunate. It ought not on that account, however,
be neglected, and I have judged that it would be neither
useless nor uninteresting to present a sketch of it to society,
which has aided, in no small degree, to advance the character of our profession. It will serve to contrast the past
with the present state of our art, and at the same time recall
to our grateful remembrance the memory of many distinguished men, who, amid numerous discouragements, did
much to elevate and adorn it.

As may naturally be presumed, in a country circum-
stanced as the American colonies were for a long period
after their original settlement, the medical profession continued for a succession of years in a low and degraded condition. In point of respectability, it undoubtedly stood
lower than either the legal or theological professions. The
religious difficulties in England had filled the ranks of the
latter with men of learning, talents and piety—while the
offices of honor and emolument under the crown, offered
allurements sufficiently powerful, to induce many who were
distinguished in the law, to emigrate to this western world.
With medicine it was far otherwise. It is only in populous
towns and cities that our art can flourish, and the wilds of
America, however fragrant they might be with the spirit of
freedom, offered no attractions to the medical men of the
old world. The advantages attending an emigration were
too distant and precarious to warrant such a step; and accordingly for a long time, with some few exceptions, none
but those who had failed to attain respectability or employment at home, would venture on so dangerous an experiment. Nor were the young native physicians for a long time
calculated to remedy the evil. To become a well qualified

physician, requires a course of study and a variety of observation which was not to be obtained in any of the colonies. There were neither lectures nor hospitals which could be resorted to, while the great expense attending a foreign education put it out of the power of all, except a favored few, to avail themselves of the only means of becoming regularly instructed. Under such circumstances it was not to have been expected, for a long series of years after the first settlement of the country, that our profession would be at all distinguished for character or knowledge. The progress of civilization, an augmenting population, together with the increasing facilities of European communication, tended gradually to meliorate this condition of things, and for many years preceding the revolution, medicine could boast of not a few names who shed a lustre upon the profession to which they belonged.

With these preliminary remarks, I propose to give a brief sketch of the state of medicine in this country anterior to the revolution, and, for the sake of convenience, shall consider it under the three divisions of *medical practice, medical literature* and *medical institutions*.

Chapter Two

MEDICAL PRACTICE

THE EARLIEST PRACTITIONERS OF MEDICINE IN THIS country appear to have been the clergy—this was at least the case in New England, where, for several years after the first settlement of the colony, the functions of the physician and divine were performed by the same individual. This combination has not been uncommon in the history of the world. In the early dawn of medicine, the priests of Egypt and Greece collected and preserved what was known of the healing art, and in the infancy of every country the same association will probably be found to exist. Nor is it, by any means, an unnatural one. Physical and moral evil are so intimately connected that those who are administering relief to the one, cannot be regardless of the other. Hence, in the absence of the regular physician, the priest appears to be his most proper representative. Besides this, the character of the first emigrants, and the high tone of religious feeling which drove them for an asylum to this western world, continued for a long time to give a preponderating influence to the clergy, in all the secular as well as religious concerns of the colony. In the annals of the first colonists, accordingly, will be found the names of several clergymen who practiced the healing art. These men were not, as might perhaps be inferred, mere empirics. On the contrary, they were by no means unqualified to practice medicine. For several years, previously to their leaving

England, and anticipating the loss of their situations as
clergymen, many of them had turned their attention to the
study of medicine, and for upwards of a century after the
settlement of New England, numbers of the native clergy
were continually educated to both professions. Altogether
they were a highly respectable class of men. Besides being
good divines, they were skilled in the medical learning of
the day, and many of them appear to have been good practical physicians.* Besides the clergy, some of the first governors of the eastern colonies also practised physic. Two of
them, of the name of Winthrop, appear to have been particularly celebrated. One of them was governor of Massachusetts, the other of Connecticut and New Haven. Of the latter, Cotton Mather says: "he was furnished with *noble medi-*

* One of the last of this class of men, at least of any eminence,
was the *Rev. Jared Elliot.* He was born in 1685 and died in 1763.
He was a graduate of Yale College, and from 1709 until his death
was minister at Killingworth in Connecticut. He published several
sermons and was so devoted to his clerical duties, that it is said
that for "forty successive years in the course of his ministry, he
never omitted preaching either at home or abroad on the Lord's
day." He was the most eminent physician of his day in Connecticut.
He appears to have read Hippocrates, Galen, Aretaeus, Celsus, &c.,
in their original languages, and he was so skilful in his management
of Chronic diseases especially, that he was frequently called in con-
sultation to Boston, Newport and other places. Besides this he was
not inattentive to matters of science and philosophy. He was the
correspondent of Bishop Berkeley and Dr. Franklin, and in "the
year 1761 received from a society in London a Gold medal, as a
premium for his discovery for extracting iron from black sand." He
is also said to have introduced the white Mulberry into Connecticut,
and with it the Silk worm and published a treatise on the subject.
In fine, he was a man eminent for his piety—his learning and skill
in medicine, and his philanthropy. *See Eliot's Biographical Diction-
ary, and Thacher's Medical Biography.*

cines, which he most charitably and generously gave away upon all occasions."* He was a member of the Royal Society of London, and some of his communications are to be found in their transactions. Amid such practice, however, as this must necessarily have been, it is easy to conceive that nothing could be done to improve the state of medicine, and that the greatest facilities must speedily have been offered for succesful imposition upon the credulity of the public. This supposition is fully confirmed by the fact that so early as the year 1649, the following law was passed in Massachusetts, evidently intended to correct existing abuses.

"Forasmuch as the law of God allows no man to impair the life or limb of any person but in a judicial way:

"It is therefore ordered, that no person or persons whatsoever, employed at any time about the bodies of men, women, or children, for preservation of life or health, as chirurgions, midwives, physicians or others, presume to exercise or put forth any act contrary to the known or approved rules of art, in each mystery and occupation, nor exercise any force, violence or cruelty, upon, or towards the body of any whether young or old, (no, not in the most difficult and desperate cases,) without the advice and consent of such as are skillful in the same art, (if any such may be had,) or at least of some of the wisest and gravest there present, and consent of the patient or patients, if they be *mentis compotes,* much less contrary to such advice and consent, upon such severe punishment as the nature of the fact may deserve; which Law, nevertheless, is not intended to discourage any from all lawful use of their skill, but rather to encourage and direct them in the right use thereof, and inhibit and restrain the presumptuous arrogancy of such as

* Magnalia Christi Americana, or the Ecclesiastical history of New England, from 1620 to 1698. Fol. p. 19. London, 1702.

through prefidence of their own skill, or any other sinister respects, dare boldly attempt to exercise any violence upon or towards the bodies of young or old, one or other to the prejudice or hazard of the life or limb of man, woman, or child."*

This appears to have been the very first attempt of the civil authority, in any of the colonies to put a restraint upon those who pretended to the practice of physic. Salutary as this law may have been, in some respects, it afforded but a slender protection against the existing deficiencies in the profession. It made no provision for the education of medical men, and it established no test of their qualifications.

The State of New York, I believe is entitled to the honor of adopting the first effectual measures for regulating the practice of medicine. This was not, however, until so late a period as 1760, when the General Assembly of the Province ordained that "no person whatsoever should practice as a physician or surgeon, in the city of New York, before he shall have been examined in physic or surgery, and approved of and admitted by one of his majesty's council, the judges of the supreme court, the king's attorney general, and the mayor of the city of New York, for the time being, or by any three or more of them, taking to their assistance for such examinations such proper person or persons as they in their discretion shall think fit." If the person so examined was approved, a certificate was given, allowing him to practice physic or surgery, or both, throughout the province. In case of non-compliance, the penalty was a fine of five pounds.†

* An act respecting chirurgions, midwives, and physicians. See ancient charters and laws of Massachusetts Bay. p. 76, 7.

† See Appendix A.

In 1772 a similar law was adopted in New Jersey.‡ These examples were not imitated in the other colonies, where the practice continued unrestrained, and physicians were responsible to no authority for mal-practice. In Connecticut an attempt was indeed made to effect a reformation in this respect, but so strong was the current of prejudice against the measure, that it completely failed.§ As far as my investigations have extended, the foregoing is all that was done, or even attempted by the constituted authorities, in behalf of our profession, previous to the revolution; and it shows conclusively how little its present respectability is owing either to the colonial governments, or to the mother country.

During the period embraced in this sketch, the division of practice into distinct departments, so generally adopted in Europe, was not recognized in this country. Both physic and surgery were practised by the same individuals; besides this, it was the general custom for physicians to prepare and compound their own medicines. In the year 1765, Dr. John Morgan, a distinguished physician of Philadelphia, endeavored to introduce a change into the existing mode of practice, by recommending a separation of it into the three branches of physic, surgery and pharmacy, and appropriating each of these departments to a separate class of practitioners. Having spent several years of his life in the acquisition of professional knowledge in countries where he had seen the practical operation of this system, he became deeply impressed with the importance of it to improve the character of the profession at home. On his return, he accordingly, not merely recommended it in a discourse which he published, but adopted it in his own practice. Although in every

‡ See Appendix B.
§ See Appendix C.

respect fully accomplished, he consequently declined in engaging in any surgical operations, and confined himself entirely to medicine.* Whatever may be thought of the general utility or propriety of such a plan, it was undoubtedly at that early period somewhat premature, and probably did not meet with much encouragement.

Until about the middle of the last century, midwifery was exclusively in the hands of females, and physicians were called in only in preternatural and tedious cases. According to Dr. Bartlett, of Massachusetts, Dr. James Lloyd was the first systematic practitioner in midwifery in that section of the United States. He had enjoyed the instructions of Warner, Sharp, Smellie and Hunter, of London, in 1753, and in the following year settled in Boston.† In 1756, Dr. William Shippen, jr., on his return from Europe, commenced the same branch of professional business in Philadelphia; and although at this period physicians were scarcely ever employed in natural labor, it is stated by his biographer, Dr. Wistar, that he did away completely with this prejudice, and in the course of a few years was fully occupied.‡

* "A discourse upon the institution of medical societies in America; delivered at a public anniversary commencement, held in the college of Philadelphia, May 30 and 31, 1765; with a preface containing among other things, the author's apology for attempting to introduce the regular mode of practising physic in Philadelphia. By JNO. MORGAN, M.D., Fellow of the Royal Society at London; correspondent of the Royal Academy of Surgery in Paris; member of the Arcadian Belles Lettres Society at Rome; Licentiate of the Royal College of Physicians in London and Edinburgh, and Professor of the Theory of Practice and Medicine in the College of Philadelphia. Philadelphia, 1765. p. 63."

† Medical Communications and Dissertations of the Mass. Medical Society, vol. 2, p. 244.

‡ Eulogium on Dr. William Shippen. By Caspar Wistar, M. D. Philadelphia, 1818, p. 31.

These are the two first physicians employed as regular accoucheurs in this country, of whom we have any notice; and they deserve especial commendation, as having led the way in overcoming deep-rooted prejudices, and in transferring to the profession, from the hands of ignorant and uneducated females, the practice of a difficult and delicate art.

From the connection subsisting between the mother country and the colonies, as may naturally be presumed, the same doctrines prevailed in both, and the practice was essentially the same. At the beginning of the eighteenth century the celebrated Boerhaave commenced his career. Gifted with every endowment natural and acquired—a mind powerful and generalizing—a fascinating eloquence—learning the most varied and profound, and a character radiant with every virtue, this great man was eminently qualified to take the foremost lead in the medical world. Not merely the age in which he lived bowed at once to the supremacy of his genius, but his doctrines continued to control the opinions and practice of medical men during the larger portion of a whole century. The leading feature in the system of this distinguished theorist, was the great and undue importance which he gave to the fluids in the production of disease. These, according to him, became variously changed, not merely in their physical properties but in their chemical composition. They became morbidly thick or thin, while they were contaminated by acid and alkaline acrimonies, and various other morbific matters. To such conditions of the fluids diseases were attributed; and medicines were supposed to act by counteracting and changing them. Such were the doctrines prevalent in the old world during the last century. Their influence was no less undisputed in this country, and the general practice was modified by them. In the management of diseases, medicines were accordingly given with the view of thinning or incrassating the blood, and altering its qualities. Much confidence was placed in the powers of nature, and the results of critical days watched with the greatest anxiety. On these, it was supposed that the *materies morbi* was discharged, and thus the relief of the patient effected. This matter was looked for chiefly in the urine, and according to Dr. Rush, "glasses to retain it were a necessary part of the furniture of every sick room."* In the treatment of fevers, sudorific medicines were principally resorted to, and to aid their operation, and to facilitate the elimination of the morbific matter, the supposed cause of disease, patients were confined to their beds, and cool air denied them in the most rigid manner. Bleeding was not a general remedy in fever. In yellow fever, so far as we can judge from the opinions of a single individual, it was considered of doubtful and even dangerous tendency.

Dr. John Mitchell, a distinguished physician of Virginia, in his account of the yellow fever which prevailed there in the years 1737, '41 and '42, in speaking of this subject, says, "plentiful bleeding is a means commonly found most effectual to obtain this end, (i.e. to ward off local inflammation) in the benign inflammatory fevers; but we cannot apply this most effectual remedy in this disease, because it evacuates only or chiefly the red globules of the blood, which, as we see by its state, taken notice of above, are in too small a proportion already; and bleeding further breaks the texture of the blood, which above all things is to be avoided in this disease; for after plentiful bleeding, the pulse sinks, or at least is so low and feeble about the state of the disease as to prove of dangerous consequences; which some instances I have known seem to confirm."† He did not, however, dis-

* Rush's Obs. and Inqs., vol. 4, p. 396.
† American Medical and Philosophical Register, vol. 4, p. 198.

card bleeding altogether. In small quantities he found it serviceable to prepare the system for other evacuations. The remedies which he principally relied on were sudorifics, but more especially cathartics. Upon the importance of this latter class of remedies, he dwells with peculiar urgency, and many of his views are characterized by great good sense and practical acumen. It was entirely by the observations and suggestions of this physician, that Dr. Rush, as he himself frankly acknowledges, was afterwards led to the free use of purgatives in the yellow fever of 1793.

In relation to yellow fever, the prevalent opinion at this period was, that it was a contagious disease. Both Drs. Mitchell* of Virginia, and Lining of Charleston, express decided opinions on this subject.† Dr. Lining, too, expresses the belief, that like small pox and measles, it does not attack

* Dr. Mitchell defines the disease in the following terms: "This distemper may be defined to be a pestilential fever, proceeding from a *contagious miasma sui generis,* which inflames the stomach and adjacent viscera, obstructs the biliary ducts, and dissolves the adipose humours; to which generally succeeds an effusion of a bilious, or other yellow humour upon the external or internal surface of the body, unless prevented by some other means." (Medical and Philo. Reg., vol. 4, p. 182.)

† Dr. Lining says, "this fever does not seem to take its origin from any particular constitution of the weather, independent of *infectious miasmata.*" Again he says, "that this is really an *infectious* disease, seems plain, not only from this, that almost all the nurses catched and died of it, but likewise, as soon as it appeared in town, it soon invaded new comers, &c." At the same time he states a fact which overthrows altogether his doctrine of contagion; it is this, "although the infection was spread with great celerity through the town, yet, if any from the country received it in town, and sicked on their return home, the infection spread no farther, *not even so much as to one in the same house.*" (Edinburgh Essays and Observations, vol. 2, p. 407.)

the second time.‡ It is hardly necessary to state, that the accurate and extended observations of more recent times have completely disproved both these positions. Indeed, if there be any one point in medicine which may now be looked upon as *settled,* it is that the yellow fever is not a contagious disease; and numerous observations incontestibly show that it may assail the human constitution a second time.

According to Dr. Rush, in his account of the state of medicine between the years 1760 and 1766, blood letting was used plentifully in pleurisies and rheumatisms, but sparingly in all other diseases;§ a practice, it must be admitted, much more judicious and safe, to say the least, than the indiscriminate and sanguinary practice which was afterwards adopted by this distinguished theorist. At this period, according to the same authority, some of the most potent and useful articles of the Materia Medica were but partially exhibited, owing to the prejudices of the public, and in some measure to the fears of the physician. Among them were the Peruvian bark and opium, both of which it was frequently necessary to disguise by admixture with other

‡ "The subjects which were susceptible of this fever were both sexes of the white color, especially strangers lately arrived from cold climates, Indians, mistees, mulattoes, of all ages, excepting young children, and of those *only such as had formerly escaped the infection. And indeed it is a great happiness that our constitutions undergo such alterations in the small pox, measles, and yellow fever, as forever afterwards secure us from a second attack of those diseases."* He then adds an interesting fact concerning the negro. "There is something very singular in the constitution of the negroes, which renders them not liable to this fever; for, though many of these were as much exposed as the nurses to the infection, yet I never knew one instance of this fever amongst them; though they are equally subject with the white people to the *bilious* fever."— Edin. Essays and Obs., vol. 2, p. 408.

§ Observations and Inquiries, vol. 4, p. 396.

medicines. Blisters were generally used, but their application was confined to the last stages of fevers. Dr. Rush says,
"wine was given sparingly even in the lowest stages of what
were then called putrid and nervous fevers."* Nevertheless,
I find that so early as 1746 the liberal use of wine in typhus
fever was recommended by that distinguished physician,
Dr. Colden, lieutenant governor of the colony of New York.
In the year just mentioned, a fever of this description prevailed epidemically at Albany, and in many cases proved
fatal. "It had the appearance of a remittent, with frequent
low pulse, except in the paroxysms, when it was high; a de-
jection of spirits, great restlessness, an entire prostration of
appetite, clammy sweats of a rancid prutrescent smell." By
the physicians of the place, it had been treated as an inter-
mittent, but without success. By the advice of Dr. Colden,
Madeira wine, to the extent of a wine glass full every four
or five hours, was ordered, and with the happiest effects.
One patient who recovered, drank a gallon in a few days. In
all those cases the wine was given in the last stages of disease.†

Dr. Chalmers too, of South Carolina, who practised at
the period alluded to by Dr. Rush, in speaking of the
"Putrid bilious fever," recommends the use of wine, in the
most unequivocal manner. "In the bilious fever we now
speak of," says he "the use of wine is indispensably necessary; nor can the quantity of it be assigned; for the sighing
and redoubled respiration, the excessive languor, mutter-
ing low sort of delirium, and want of heat in the extreme
parts, together with a clamminess on the backs of the hands,
or more general cold sweats, plainly point out the great
want of excitement in the vital and animal functions. Red

* Observations and Inquiries, vol. 4, p. 399.
† London Medical Observat, and Inquiries, vol. 1, p. 215.

port wine may therefore be given, punch and other spirituous and vinous fermented liquors of the greatest strength, ought to be liberally allowed in these cases, *with this only proviso,* that the head be not too much affected thereby."‡

Although the physicians in the colonies generally followed the prevalent practice of the mother country, yet they are entitled to the credit of originating some modes of practice of great value. The most important of these is the application of mercury in the treatment of inflammatory complaints. This practice took its origin as far back as the year 1736, and the credit of originality is generally conceded to Dr. Douglass, a physician of Boston, by whom it was used in the angina maligna which prevailed extensively over the colonies at that period, and committed the most dreadful ravages.* By Dr. James Ogden, a respectable physician of Long Island, this practice was extensively applied in the same disease about the year 1749.† The preparation of mercury which was used was calomel. In consequnce of the success which attended the use of this remedy in this disease, it was shortly after resorted to in other inflammatory complaints; and about the middle of the last century, it was in common use in this country in pleurisy, pneumonia, rheumatism, and others of the phlegmasiae. I am aware that the credit of this practice is claimed elsewhere;§ but there can

‡ On the climate and diseases of South Carolina, vol. 1, p. 166.
* New England Journal of Medicine, vol. 14, p. 4.
† New York Med. Repository, vol. 5, p. 97.
§ Dr. John Armstrong, in his work on Typhus, gives the sole credit of this practice to Dr. Robert Hamilton of Lynn Regis. In another place, I have shown the incorrectness of this statement. (See Infant Therapeutics.) From the account of Dr. Hamilton himself, it appears that his attention was not called to the practice until the year 1764; whereas it had been in very general use in this country many years before.

be no doubt that in its origin it is exclusively American, and that to our colonial physicians the world is indebted for one of the greatest improvements ever made in practical medicine.

Among the events which characterized the history of our colonial medicine, the most remarkable, and certainly the most exciting, were those which attended the introduction of the practice of inoculation for the small pox. This was first introduced into this country in the year 1721; and it is to a clergyman, Dr. Cotton Mather, that the honor belongs of having first recommended it. During this year the small pox raged in Boston with unparalleled fury and fatality. Dr. Mather having read, in the transactions of the Royal Society of London, an account of a new mode of mitigating the violence of the disease by inoculation, as practised in Turkey, communicated it to the physicians of the place, and urged their adoption of it. With the exception of one individual, it was unanimously opposed by the faculty. This individual was Dr. Zabdiel Boylston, who, with the confidence of an honest and enlightened mind, commenced his operations upon his own children and servants.* The controversies which ensued were of the most ferocious and disreputable character. Such was the tempest

* The first experiments by Boylston were made on the 27th June, 1721, on his own son, thirteen years of age, and two blacks in his own family, one of thirty-six and the other two years of age, and all with success. During the prevalence of the small pox in that and the following year, he inoculated with his own hand two hundred and forty-seven of both sexes, from nine months to sixty-seven years of age. Thirty-nine were inoculated by other physicians after the tumult had somewhat subsided, making in all two hundred and eighty-six, of whom only six died. During the same period, 5,759 had taken the natural small pox, 844 of whom had died. See Thacher's Medical Biography, p. 163.

of popular indignation raised against the practice, chiefly by the inflammatory conduct of the physicians, at the head of whom was Dr. Douglass, that both Drs. Mather and Boylston were in danger of losing their lives. Passion and prejudice on the one side were, however, met by decision and success on the other; and inoculation, defended by almost all the clergy, many of whom preached and wrote in its defence, soon triumphed over opposition, and became prevalent in Boston and the neighboring towns. From thence it was introduced into the other colonies, and although uniformly resisted at first, the public mind became gradually reconciled to it. So early as 1738, it was practised in Charleston, S. C., during the epidemic small pox which then prevailed there. In 1759 it was generally adopted in Philadelphia, where its dissemination was very much facilitated by a defence and recommendation of it by Dr. Redman. The true merit of Dr. Boylston, in relation to the introduction of inoculation, will not be appreciated unless it is stated that at this time the practice had only just found its way into Europe. By a singular coincidence, the first case of inoculation in Europe took place in England in April, 1721, only two months before the first experiment of Dr. Boylston, and entirely without his knowledge. This was the case of the daughter of Lady Wortley Montague. This celebrated female, during her residence in Constantinople, having become acquainted with the safety of the practice, had her son inoculated, and on her return to England, her daughter was subjected to the same operation, and with perfect safety.† This led the way to the speedy diffusion of the practice in England, as the experiments of Boylston did in this country. It is gratifying to know, that although opposed and

† The history of the inoculation of the small pox, &c. By William Woodville, M. D., vol. 1, p. 85.

slandered at home, this eminent physician was appreciated abroad. In 1725 he visited England, and was received with the highest favor and attention by the most distinguished characters in the nation, and even by royalty itself. He was elected a fellow of the Royal Society, being the first instance in which that honor was conferred upon an American.

Among the practices peculiar to the colonies, was the administration of mercury as a preparative to inoculation. By the illustrious Boerhaave, it had before been suggested that mercury would prove an antidote to small pox; and from him, no doubt, the hint was taken. In 1724, Dr. Huxham also recommended calomel, not merely in the natural small pox, but also when inoculated.† It was only in the colonies, however, that the practice was tried on a large scale; and an interesting account of its effects has been left us by Dr. Benjamin Gale, of Connecticut, in a paper published in the Philosophical Transactions for 1765. The credit of the practice is given by him to Dr. Thomas, of Virginia, and Dr. Munson, of Long Island, by whom it was established in 1745. According to the statements of Dr. Gale, it appears that the deaths from the natural small pox, before inoculation was introduced into New England, averaged 1 in 7 or 8; when inoculation was introduced, the deaths amounted to 1 in 30. By improvements and proper precautions, they were reduced to 1 in 80 to 100; and finally, by preparing the system by the previous use of mercury, the deaths were only 1 in 800 or 1000.*

For the early and prompt investigation, as well as the

† Woodville's History of Inoculation, vol. 1, p. 342.

* Historical Memoirs, relating to the practice of Inoculation for the Small pox, in the British American Provinces, particularly in New England. By Benjamin Gale. See Philosophical Transactions, abridged, vol. 12, p. 229.

sound and original views which they advanced in relation to the pathology and treatment of that acute and now well-known disease, croup, our colonial physicians are entitled to the highest applause. Although not unknown or unnoticed previously, the credit is generally conceded to Dr. Home, of Edinburgh, of having given the first full description of this disease. This appeared in 1765. In 1771, Dr. Crawford published his "Disquisitio Inauguralis de Cynanche Stridula;" and in 1788 appeared the elaborate work of Michaelis of Gottingen, entitled "Dissertatio Inauguralis de Angina Polyposa sive membranacea." These were all the foreign publications which had appeared on this interesting subject. Between the years 1770 and 1781, in this country, Drs. Rush, S. Bard, Chalmers, Middleton and Bayley, all published in relation to it, and by them especially the two latter, more correct views were enforced than had been entertained by Home and others. Contrary to the opinion of Home, that the secretion of mucus on the inside of the trachea was the cause of the disease, Dr. Bayley established the fact that the disease was an inflammation of the mucous membrane of the trachea, and that the effusion and false membrane were the consequences of this inflammation. Based upon the idea that it was an acute and rapid inflammation, the treatment recommended was of the most decided character. Blood-letting *ad deliquium*—the free use of tartar emetic, at first to produce vomiting, and then to keep up nausea, together with the free use of calomel, were all originally recommended by them, although the credit of every one of them has since been claimed by others.* In

---

* As a sample of the manner in which practices originating in this country, are appropriated abroad, not from design, but ignorance, the following may be adduced. Dr. Stokes, in his recent and invaluable treatise on diseases of the chest, in speaking of tartar

determining the true nature of this disease, as well as the treatment most efficacious, the merit of Bayley stands pre-eminent, and the tract which he has left upon this subject, is sufficient of itself to establish his reputation as an original observer and an able and accomplished practitioner.†

If we may believe the authority of Dr. Douglass, who wrote about the year 1753, and of Smith, the historian of New York, the general character of the profession could not have been very elevated, and quackery must have flourished in great perfection.‡ Douglass speaks of it in the following terms: "In general, the physical practice in our colonies is so perniciously bad, that excepting in surgery, and some very acute cases, it is better to let nature, under a proper regimen, take her course, than to trust to the honesty and sagacity of the practitioner; our American practitioners are so rash and officious, the saying in the apocrypha, (38 and 15,) may with much propriety be applied to them. *"He that sinneth before his Maker, let him fall into the hands of the physician!* Frequently, there is more danger from the physician than from the distemper. Our practition-

emetic in croup, holds the following language: "For the introduction of this inestimable remedy in the treatment of the croup, the science is indebted to Dr. Cheyne. In his Essay on Cyanche Trachealis, published in Edinburgh in 1801, we find the treatment recommended; and it is no small evidence in its favor, that in the year 1832, after an experience greater than falls to the lot of most men, the opinions of this philosophical investigator of disease have remained unaltered. How changed would be the character of medicine, if, in support of many of our remedies, there could be brought forward such evidence, and such an advocate." P. 144, Amer. Ed. Dr. Bayley recommended and used the same remedy, in the same way, and with the same objects in view, a quarter of a century before.

† Cases of Angina Trachealis, with the mode of cure: in a letter to William Hunter, M. D., &c. By Richard Bayley, Surgeon. Printed,

ers deal much in quackery and quackish medicines, as requiring no labor of thought or composition, and highly recommended in the London quack bills, (in which all the reading of many of our practitioners consists,) inadvertently encouraged by patents for the benefit of certain fees to some offices, but to the very great damage of the subject." "In the most trifling cases, they use a routine of practice. When I first arrived in New England, I asked a most noted facetious practitioner what was their general method of practice; he told me their practice was very uniform: bleeding, vomiting, blistering, purging, anodynes, &c.; if the illness continued, there was *repetendi,* and finally *murderandi;* nature was never to be consulted or allowed to have any concern in the affair: What Sydenham well observes is the case with our practitioners: Aeger nimia medici diligentia ad plures migret."§

New York, 1781. For the purpose of showing the views of Bayley in relation to the nature and cure of this disease, I shall quote the following from his paper: "When the Angina Trachealis is theoretically considered, there will probably be formed, (as is generally the case when facts are not ascertained) opinions as various as the information and different faculties of men may suggest. I am induced to adopt the following: That the larynx, aspera arteria, and bronchial pipes, have one common membrane, which, we are informed by injection, consists of little more than an infinity of blood-vessels, and consequently liable to *inflammation,* as all vascular parts are. An increased action of these vessels (as in pleuritic and puerperal fevers) occasions a preternatural secretion of lymph, which from the ingress and egress of the air becomes condensed, and assumes the appearance of a membrane, and its compactness will depend upon the age and habit of the patient and the state of the atmosphere.

"The common opinion is, that those who die of this complaint are suffocated by the membrane's closing the wind pipe. Another more respectable opinion is, that a spasm of the muscles of the larynx closes the scene. The circumstances which precede *death* in

Smith, who wrote in 1758, says, "few physicians among us are eminent for their skill. Quacks abound like locusts in Egypt, and too many have recommended to a full practice and profitable subsistence. This is the less to be wondered at, as the profession is under no kind of regulation. Loud as the call is, to our shame be it remembered, we have no law to protect the lives of the King's subjects, from the malpractice of pretenders. Any man, at his pleasure, sets up for physician, apothecary and chirurgeon. No candidates are either examined or licensed, or were sworn to fair practice."**

The following picture of the state of physic in New York in 1767, is given by a competent witness, Dr. Middleton. It is by no means flattering either to the public or to the profession.

"Yet many, too many, are the instances, even in this place, of men, otherwise valuable for their penetration and good sense, who have given up their own judgments to the opinions of the credulous vulgar; and joining in the belief of *nostrums,* or *secret cures,* have countenanced, and even employed the most obscure and superficial traders in physic.

this disease, compared with those appearances which have regularly taken place in the cases which I have seen *successfully* treated, sufficiently explain the cause of the patient's death from the laws of the blood's circulation. To preserve the healthful state of an animal, it is necessary that the whole mass of blood should circulate through the lungs in a given time, and the free admission and expulsion of air contributes to this regular process; the change, also, which gradually takes place in the lungs, seems more directly to account for the swelled face, tumid jugulars and the full staring eyes, which are symptoms that accompany the progress of this complaint; and add to this, the larynx, aspera arteria and bronchia have been found pervious in every subject I have dissected, while the ramifications have been as regularly filled with a glairy mucus.

While the practitioner of modesty and real merit, conscious of his own integrity and knowledge, and scorning the little arts of such licensed freebooters and secret homicides, or to stoop to the unreasonable humors of petulance of every employer, has often had very circumscribed practice; or has been abandoned in favor of some ignorant or mercenary sycophant. This conduct in such men will ever discourage genuine worth, and the prospect of farther discoveries in that useful profession; which in all times, and among all polite nations, has ever been esteemed honorable, and worthy of men of the first rank and learning.

"Such being the state of physic here, what wonder is it that this city should be pestered in so remarkable a manner with the needy outcasts of other places, in the character of doctors; or that this profession, of all others, should be the receptacle and resource for the refuse of every other trade and employment? The wonder indeed is, that we should be such dupes to their effrontery as to employ them, or buy their pernicious compositions; not that they should frequent

"From what precedes, it is obvious that the angina trachaelis is considered as an *inflammatory disease* the treatment of which must vary in every degree, according to its violence: and though the common antiphlogistic treatment will in some cases relieve, if early applied, yet the most desperate may yield to *repeated bleedings ad deliquium* from the jugulars, the free use of *tartar emetic* and other evacuants, with *a large blister* covering the larynx and aspera arteria, while the mucus filling up the ramifications of the bronchla may be emptied by the action of vomiting." See New York Medical Repository, vol. 14, p. 346. Although not published until the year 1781, the paper of Bayley contains the results of his observations and practice for a number of years previously.

‡History of New York, by William Smith, A. M. p. 326.

§ A Summary, historical and political, of the first planting, profession, improvements, and present state of the British Settlements in North America. By William Douglass, M.D. Boston, V. 2, p. 352.

so beneficial a market. So amazingly easy of belief are some people in these miracle-mongers, that, as if there was something creative in the name of Doctor, seldom any other test of their skill is required than their assuming that title; so that this appellation, with a competent presence of mind and a string of ready-coined cures, carefully propagated by such as find their account in carrying on the cheat, have seldom failed in procuring traffic in New York."*

Virginia too seems to have been overrun with empirics, who by their inordinate charges annoyed the inhabitants of the Colony so much that the General Assembly passed various acts in 1639, 1661 and 1736, regulating the fees they should receive. In doing this the Assembly made a just distinction between the ordinary practitioners and those who had received a regular education, and had received a diploma from some university.†

That in a state of society where the means of medical education were so scanty, and where no laws existed to regulate the profession or restrain admission into ranks, quack-

** "The necessity of regulating the practice of physic, and a plan for that purpose, were strongly recommended by the authors of the Independent Reflector, in 1753, when the city of New York alone boasted the honor of having above forty gentlemen of that faculty." History of New York from the first discovery to the year 1732. By William Smith, A. M., p. 326.

* A Medical Discourse, or an Historical Inquiry into the Ancient and Present State of Medicine; the substance of which was delivered at the opening of the Medical School in the city of New York. By PETER MIDDLETON, M.D., and Professor of the Theory of Physic in King's College.

'Est quoddam prod re tenui.'—HOR.
'Curentnr dubii medicis majoribus aegri.'—JUV.
Printed by desire. New York: Printed by Hugh Gaine, in Hanover Square, 1769. p. 63, 4.

† See Appendix, D.

ery should be very rife, is certainly by no means singular. It would be unjust, however, to suppose that it is peculiar to such a state of society, or even that it prevailed to a greater extent than it does in the present day. Mortifying as it is, it is, nevertheless a fact, that it is peculiar to no particular age, or country, or state of society. It has existed from the earliest periods, and will continue to exist as long as human beings are found upon the face of the earth. The rude savage and the polished citizen are equally its victims, and civilization and refinement only render its forms more complicated and insidious. At no period in the history of this country, it may safely be asserted, has empiricism flourished to the same fearful extent as at the present time, notwithstanding our boasted improvements in other respects. Assuming a thousand different disguises, it is in many high places in our country, sapping the very honor of the profession, and corrupting it to the core. Notwithstanding the prevalence of quackery in the colonies, it does not appear that the well educated part of the profession lent it any countenance, and it would be well if the same could be said in the present day. A recollection of these facts should therefore moderate somewhat the severity of our judgment in relation to the state of our colonial medicine, at the same time that it should excite us to renewed diligence in endeavoring, if possible, to correct existing abuses.

Chapter Three

MEDICAL LITERATURE

I COME NEXT TO TAKE A BRIEF NOTICE OF THE STATE OF medical literature previous to the revolution. Although not abounding in materials of very high interest or importance, the medical literature of this period is by no means contemptible. In forming a judgment in relation to it, we should recollect the circumstances in which the American physician was placed, and the slender inducements which were held out to undertake the labors of authorship. The two great motives which induce men, in any age, to write— the love of literary distinction, and the hope of pecuniary gain, then exercised but a feeble and limited influence; and accordingly, the colonial physicians only turned authors on some special emergency of public duty, or for the purpose of promulgating and enforcing some new and useful mode of practice. The capabilities of our early physicians, therefore, ought to be judged of, not so much by the quantity, as by the quality, of the productions which they have left us, and an impartial review of them will show us that they do not suffer by a comparison with the productions of their European brethren at the same period. Some of them were not thought unworthy of being published in the Transactions of the Royal Society, while others found a place in the publications of the learned medical associations of the day, in the mother country.

A brief review of what appeared in the colonies, will be, not merely interesting, as a matter of historical record, but will furnish the best evidence of the general drift and progress of medical mind during this period.

The earliest medical publications appeared in *Massachusetts*, and were called forth by the prevalence of epidemic diseases, and the first appears to have been a tract by Thomas Thatcher, a clergyman and physician of Massachusetts. It was entitled "A Brief Guide in the Small Pox and Measles," and was published in the year 1677. Cotton Mather, in his Magnalia, gives the life of this person, and represents him as a man of learning and ingenuity.*

In 1721, *Benjamin Colman,* a minister of Boston, printed a small pamphlet entitled—"Some Account of the New Method of Receiving the Small Pox, by Ingrafting or Inoculating;" in which he defends the practice of inoculation, which had just been introduced by Dr. Boylston.

Five years after this, Dr. *Boylston,* while on his visit to England, published there, at the request of the Royal Society, "An Historical Account of the Small Pox, inoculated in New-England." In the following year it was reprinted in Boston.

In addition to the above may be mentioned the names of Thomas Howard and Nathaniel Williams, both of whom were clergymen as well as physicians. The former wrote

* He was born in England in 1620, and came to this country in 1635. He was a man of great learning, especially in the oriental languages. He published a Hebrew Lexicon, and was skilled in the Arabic. According to Dr. Mather, he was a "great logician; he understood mechanism in theory and practice, and would make all kinds of clock work to admiration." He was eminent, not merely as a divine, but as a physician, and served in both capacities, first at Weymouth and then in Boston. See *Thacher's Medical Biography.*

a Treatise on Pharmacy, in 1732; and the latter a pamphlet "On the Method of Practice in the Small Pox in 1730."

The most voluminous writer, however, who appeared at this period, was Dr. *William Douglass.* He was a native of Scotland, and emigrated to New England about the year 1716. Although a man of talent and learning, he appears to have been of an unhappy temper of mind, to which he gave loose in many of his writings.* He was a most virulent opponent of the practice of inoculation, and did all in his power to excite popular indignation against it. Besides several publications on this subject, he has left a tract on the putrid sore throat distemper, which prevailed epidemically for several years in the colonies.† As this paper contains the only full account of a disease which attracted more than any other, the attention of our colonial physicians, it is worthy of a brief analysis. It furnishes the best description extant of the disease, and at the same time gives a good practical illustration of the views of practice at that period. The first appearance of the disease, was on the 20th of May, 1735, at Kingston an inland town of New England, about 50 miles eastward of Boston. It was vulgarly called the *"throat illness,* or a *plague in the throat."* It was here that the disease displayed itself in its greatest malignity, according to Dr. Doug-

* He is represented to have "been deficient in judgment, prudence and correct taste, he assumed the task of animadverting upon the actions and character of others, filling the newspapers with political essays, fraught with sarcastic remarks upon the magistrate, the clergy, the physicians and the people of New England." American Medical Biography &c., by James Thacher, M. D., p. 255.

† The practical history of a new epidemical eruptive miliary fever, with an angina ulcusculosa, which prevailed in New England in 1735 and '36, by WILLIAM DOUGLASS, M. D., Boston 1736. Reprinted in the New England Journal of Medicine and Surgery, vol. 14, p. 1.

lass. "Some died of a sudden or acute necrosis; but most of them by a symptomatick affection of the fauces or neck; that is by sphacelatious or corrosive ulcerations in the fauces, or by an infiltration and tumefaction in the chops and fore part of the neck, so turgid, as to bring all upon a level between the chin and sternum, occasioning a strangulation of the patient in a short time." Its first appearance in Boston was on the 20th of August. Its general character here was however much milder than in the country. In Boston, Dr. Douglass estimates the whole number attacked with the disease about 4,000, which was about one fourth of the population, and of those attacked about 1 in 35 died. In the country towns, on the contrary, one in three of the sick, in others one in four, and in scarce any fewer than one in six died. The disease assumed various forms. Generally speaking in most of the patients, along with the common symptoms of fever, such as chill, pains in various parts of the body, nausea or vomiting, the uvula and tonsils became inflamed, tumefied with white specks upon them, together with a general efflorescence, beginning in the face and spreading over the neck, chest and extremities. On the 3d or 4th day this efflorescence reached its height, after which it terminated in a general itching and scaling off of the cuticle, and at the same time the specks and sloughs in the throat were thrown off. Cases of this description, he says, if left to nature with a "warm soft regimen, had generally an easy and salutary course in six or seven days." If on the contrary they were interfered with either by a stimulating or depleting practice they were protracted or ended badly; when the case assumed a bad character, there was great prostration of strength, despondency of mind, low pulse, incessant vomitings, purgings and sweats, excessive inflammation of the tonsils producing almost strangulation, with brown or livid

specks in the fauces—ichorous discharges from the mouth
and nose, sometimes stupor &c. In these cases the eruption
on the skin was livid, alternately appearing and receding.
Many of those affected in this way, died on the sixth or
seventh day.

In the worst kind of cases the disease assumed a still
more malignant character. The patients were generally
seized suddenly; there was a sinking pain at the stomach,
extreme prostration of strength, low pulse; in some, stupor,
in others delirium; in children, convulsions; colliquative
vomiting, purging and sweats, with rapid decomposition
after death. These cases terminated fatally on the first, second, or third day, and as Dr. Douglass expresses it, "by an
irremediable necrosis of the oeconomy." Venesection, and
other evacuations, only accelerated death in these cases. In
the treatment of the disease, Dr. Douglass shows much judgment and discrimination. In the ordinary form of it he
trusted very much to nature. "In the standard kind," says he,
"when left to nature, with a warm, soft regimen, it had generally an easy and salutary course in six or seven days; but
when by a hot, cordial method—or on the other extreme, by
being too much exposed to the cold, or by officious, profuse
evacuations, nature was disturbed in her work—the distemper was protracted, or some consequential ails from an
imperfect defecation ensued."

When nature required any assistance, the remedy chiefly
relied on was *calomel.* As this was a practice, at that time
perfectly original, it may not be uninteresting to the reader
to be made acquainted with the reasons which led to the use
of this remedy. In explaining his views on this subject, Dr.
Douglass says, "any affection of the throat does frequently
produce a natural ptyalism; mercurials used with discretion
are a kind of specific in such like ulcers, or ulcuscula, and in

fact, here they moistened the throat and mouth, stopt the spreading of the ulcuscula and promoted the casting off of the sloughs; and as an accessary advantage, (the patients being mostly children,) destroyed worms: amongst all its preparations *calomel* answered best; the gentle vomiting or few stools that it occasioned in some, did not confound the natural course of the distemper. *Turbeth* proves, generally, too strong a revulsion, and the eruption is thereby too much diverted; this distemper did not well bear any other evacuations but *mercurials.*" And in other place he adds, "The despumation of this acrid inquination of the juices in our distemper, that is, its natural crisis, seems to be by the potent and salutary emunctories of the fauces and skin. In corrosive taints, v. g. venereal and others, a mercurial ptyalism and sudorific decoction of the woods answer best; this gave us the hint of promoting the tendency of nature, in our illness, by *mercurials* and gentle-breathing sweats a-bed; which with good management, seldom failed, excepting where the necrosis was irremediable from the beginning." Blood-letting, except occasionally, he condemns as exceedingly injurious. "If the fever is too high, (which however was very seldom the case,) if the patient is plethoric, or accustomed to venesection," he directs "some blood to be taken, but with discretion; if the tonsils were much inflamed, with great pain and difficulty in swallowing," he advises the jugulars to be opened. On the other hand, the hot, cordial treatment he equally condemns. In cases of great prostration of the powers of life he recommends "generous wine," and other stimulants. As a local application, to cleanse the throat and separate the slough, he advises a gargle of the tincture of aloes and myrrh. Profuse sweats and diarrhoea were checked by elix. vitriol and toasted rhubarb. In the conclusion of this essay Dr. Douglass makes some general remarks of an interesting character. Among others, he expresses the opinion that the disease was a new epidemic, not known before; that it did not depend upon any change of the seasons, as it prevailed during the whole of the year; that it did not depend upon any peculiarity of soil or climate, as it prevailed throughout the whole extent of the Colonies, from Massachusetts to South Carolina. He remarks, however, that "in damp places, as near large ponds, fresh-water rivers, woodlands and the like, it did the most execution." In addition to this he says it was not personally infectious, like the small-pox, &c., but that it "proceeded from some undiscovered quality of the air, affecting only peculiar constitutions of persons and families." No second attacks were observed, and no condition was exempt. "Europeans, West Indians, Indians, negroes, of all ages, were equally subject to it; but, as in most epidemical diseases, it affected children and the younger persons more generally." With regard to the treatment, he makes the significant remark, that *"most of those who died of the physician died by immoderate evacuations."*

The preceding is an imperfect analysis as the paper of Dr. Douglass. Although written in a quaint style, it is a most remarkable production. There can be no question that the disease described by him was the same as the scarlatina of the present day, presenting itself in the principal varieties of the simple, anginose and malignant. These he describes very accurately, and he seems to have thoroughly understood the disease in all its forms and peculiarities. His views of the treatment too, are in the main excellent, and correspond with the most enlightened experience of the present day. Confident with regard to the merits of his paper, he closes his essay with the following prophetic words. "This is a real history of the distemper as it appeared in

Boston, New England, taken clinically from the life and not copied. There is no shock or clause, but what I can vouch by real, not imaginary causes. It is founded only upon observations or phenomena that is upon the symptoms that appeared in the course of this epidemical disease; *it must therefore be of permanent truth.*"

The most elaborate work, of this author, was "A Summary, Historical and Political, of the First Planting, Progressive Improvements, and Present State of the British Settlements in North America." This was published in 1760, in two volumes, 8vo., and contains some amusing notices of the state of the profession in the colonies.

These were pretty much all the medical writers of whom Massachusetts could boast for upwards of a century and a half.

In the middle and southern colonies, medicine appears to have been cultivated with much more success than in the eastern. This may be accounted for by the fact that the former enjoyed the services of several foreign physicians, who had early emigrated thither, enriched by the best medical education which Europe could afford. It appears also to have been more common with them to send their young men to foreign universities to complete their medical studies. In addition to all this, a taste for researches in natural history began to develope itself much sooner in some of the southern colonies, and doubtless produced a salutary effect in spreading the influence of liberal sentiments. To these causes is to be attributed the early superiority of the the southern colonies more especially.

Of the colonial physicians none were more active or distinguished than those of *South Carolina*. In 1734, a native of this state, *William Bull,* obtained a degree in medicine, at the university of Leyden, and on that occasion, defended

and published an inaugural dissertation, "De Colica Picto-
num." He had studied under Boerhaave, and seems to have
commanded the respect of his associates. By the celebrated
Van Swieten, he is spoken of in his commentaries as the
very learned W. Bull.* In 1749 *John Moultrie* received the
degree of doctor in medicine, at the university of Edinburgh, and published a thesis, "De Febre Flava." He was the
first native Carolinian who obtained this honor at that university. According to Dr. Ramsay, ten other native Caro-
linians obtained the same honor, between the years 1768
and '78.† As more particularly distinguished in this section
of the country, the names of Drs. *Lining, Chalmers* and
Garden, deserves to be especially noticed. They were all
natives of Scotland, and emigrated in the earlier part of the
last century. Being men of unquestioned abilities, learning
and enterprise, they contributed greatly, both by their influence and writings, to elevate the character of the profession. To Dr. *John Lining,* we are indebted for some of the
most valuable statical experiments ever published. They
were continued throughout the whole of the year 1740. He
ascertained his weight in the morning and evening; the
weight of the food which he swallowed, and the weight of
the urine and alvine excretions ejected. The result of these
troublesome experiments was published in 1743, in the

* Hoec colica in regionibus Americae meridionalibus tam
frequens est, ut fere pro morbo endemio haberi possit; uti ab
Eruditissimo viro Gulielmo Bull, in his oris nato, et, nunc feliciter
ibi medicinam exercente, soepius audivi, qui et pulchram de hoc
morbo scripsit dissertationem inauguralem, quam de academia
Lugduno Batava defendit anno 1734. Van Swieten's Commentaries,
Vol. iii, p. 357.

† Ramsay's Review of Medicine in the 18th century. New York
Medical Repository, vol. iv. p. 398.

Transactions of the Royal Society of London.* In 1753 he published "A description of the American Yellow Fever," in a letter to the celebrated Dr. Robert Whytt, professor of medicine in the university of Edinburgh. This was the first account of this terrible disorder which had emanated from this continent, and stands to this day unrivalled for the general accuracy and minuteness of its description.†

To Dr. *Lionel Chalmers* we are also indebted for several valuable productions. In the year 1754 he communicated to the Medical Observations and Inquiries of London, a paper on the *Opisthotonos and Tetanus*. These appear to have been very prevalent at that time, in Charlestown, and Dr. Chalmers seems to have had a large experience in them. The remedies which he principally recommends are, blood-letting in the commencement, the warm bath, the free use of opium, and emollient enemata.‡ In 1768, he published "An Essay on Fevers," in which he enters into an extensive discussion of the theory of febrile diseases, and proposes a new method of treating them. Contrary to the prevalent belief of the time, Dr. Chalmers endeavors to show that the cause of the fever is not to be sought for in the fluids, but in the solids, and he considers the immediate cause to be "a spasmodic constriction of the arteries and other muscular membranes." Whatever can give much pain or stimulate the nerves so as to cause them to excite such constrictions, he thinks may bring on fever. As an inevitable

---

* Vol. xiii. p. 491. Thomson's History of the Royal Society, p. 129.

† A description of the *American Yellow Fever*, in a letter from Dr. John Lining, Physician at Charleston in South Carolina, to Robert Whytt, Professor of Medicine in the University of Edinburgh, p. 28. Edinburgh Essays and Observations V. 2, p. 404.

‡ Vol. 1, page 87.

consequence of this spasm and constriction, irregular distributions of blood take place, producing engorgements of the different viscera, and to this irregular circulation are owing all the phenomena of fever. Spasm of the extreme arteries and irregular distribution of the blood being the leading features of fever, he recommends two indications in the treatment. First, to relax the spasm—second, to relieve the internal fulness of the system; and the two agents he recommends for accomplishing these purposes are, sweating and purging. Such is a very brief account of his theory of fever, which he supports with much talent and learning. The whole work displays a compass of observation, and a power of theoretical discussion, which should have raised its author to a higher rank than he seems to hold in the lists of medical fame. To perfect originality the theory of Dr. Chalmers can lay no claim. The doctrine of spasm had been previously suggested by the celebrated Hoffman, from whom both Chalmers and Cullen doubtless borrowed it. Whether Chalmers was at all indebted to Cullen for any of his views on this subject, it is not easy to say, although it seems very improbable, the essay of Dr. Chalmers having appeared several years before the "First Lines" of Dr. Cullen were presented to the public. Besides this, Dr. Chalmers was the author of a most valuable work on the Climate and Diseases of South Carolina.* This production was the result of upwards of twenty years experience, and is worthy of especial notice, as being the first and only work we have which gives an account of the peculiar diseases of any of the colonies. It shows the author to have been a man of accurate observation —most excellent judgment and discriminating views, of the

---

* Account of the Weather and Diseases of South Carolina. By LIONEL CHALMERS, M.D., of Charles-Town, South-Carolina. London, 1776. 2 vol. 8vo. pp. 222-224.

nature and treatment of disease. It fully merits a place along side of the works of Huxham and Cleghorn. The following description of Charlestown is interesting as having been written upwards of seventy years ago.

"The white inhabitants of this town may be about five thousand five hundred; but the mortality among them cannot be exactly determined at present, no register thereof having been kept for several years. Formerly when bills of mortality were annually printed, the inhabitants then being not quite four thousand, it appeared that one in thirty-seven died yearly, or about one out of each family in the space of seven years and a half." "There are many more negroes than white people in this town and province; and those of African descent are as susceptible of all sorts of diseases as those of other color, if we except the *yellow or malignant fever* and *gout*. Besides, they are liable to particular complaints, which seem peculiar to negroes only. However, even blacks, who live in all respects, as we commonly do, are equally obnoxious to gout with white men. Births cannot be ascertained from the christenings; for children are not baptised the same year in which they are born. But it is certain they far exceed the deaths of the settled inhabitants.

The natives for the most part, rise above the middling stature, and they attain their full height sooner, than the people usually do in colder climates. In general, they are of a slender make, have pale complexions, thin, fair or brown hair, which afterwards changes to a chestnut or black color; but it seldom curls. They are forward in genius, and thought capable of receiving instruction earlier, than children in Britain commonly are; with respects to their character, they are exceedingly hospitable, and of a mild temper, which is yet not without a quick sensibility of any designed affront;

but their passions soon subside. Few live sixty years; and the bald or hoary and wrinkled appearances of old age, often show themselves at the age of thirty years; or even earlier, more especially on those who dwell in the country.

The women are in full bloom between their sixteenth and twenty-fifth year; and they very generally are well featured and genteel in person. The menses commonly begin to flow between the twelfth and fourteenth year; and that discharge ceases at different periods between the thirtieth and fiftieth year of their ages, according as constitutions vary." p. 36, 37, 8.

Of the diseases, which at that period were the most prevalent in Carolina, *gout* seems to have taken the lead. Dr. Chalmers makes the following statement on this subject. "I am persuaded, that for the number of people, the *gout* is more common in this province than in any other country, and it attacks very many in whom no hereditary taint can be traced; but youth, sprung from *gouty* parents, are sometimes seized with that disease before they are twelve years old. It is thought by some, that the reason why we are so much inclined to *arthritick* disorders, may in part be owing to the constant use that is made of by many of weak sour punch. Yet, though that sort of liquor is now much less in esteem amongst us than it formerly was, this disease is notwithstanding rather more frequent than before. But, in my opinion, it may with more probability be imputed to a bad digestion, from an *atonia* of the stomach; for that part is equally weakened with others, by the great and continued heat of our summer weather. It is indeed true, that the first English settlers of this country, suffered but little from the *gout*, though the climate must have been more sultry and damp at that time than it is at present; because, the land being now much cleared of trees and underwood, with which it was in a manner covered in those days, the *air* consequently has a freer passage through the inhabited parts of the province. But those people led a laborious life; had many hardships to encounter, and their diet was more plain and simple than that of their successors."*

Dr. Chalmers also recorded and published an important series of metrological observations at Charlestown, continued for ten years, i.e., from 1750 to 1760.†

Dr. *Alexander Garden* was another distinguished physician of Charlestown at this period. From all the accounts which we have left of him, he appears to have been a man not merely thoroughly versed in his profession, but highly accomplished in literature and general science. He was much devoted to natural history; and the transactions of the Royal Society contain several of his papers on this department. As a proof of the high estimation in which he was held, it may be mentioned, that Linnaeus, with whom he corresponded in Latin, gave the name of Gardenia (in honor of him) to "one of the most beautiful flowering shrubs in the world." He was a member of the Royal societies of Upsal and of London. The only medical production which he has left, is an account of the anthelmintic properties of the *Spigelia Marylandica,* together with a botanical description of the plant published in 1771.‡

* On the climate and diseases of South Carolina, vol. 2. p. 175, 6.

† A general table of the results of these observations may be seen in his work on Carolina, vol. 1, p. 42.

‡ An account of the Indian pink, by ALEX. GARDEN, M. D., in Charlestown, South Carolina, member of the Royal Society at Upsal, and of the Philorophical Society of Edinburgh, communicated in three letters 1764-65, and presented by Dr. Hope. Edinb. essays and observations, physical and literary, vol. 3, p. 145. For an interesting account of Dr. Garden, see Ramsay's History of South Carolina, vol. 2.

This plant grows abundantly in the low rich lands of South Carolina, and for the first knowledge of its *anthelmintic virtues,* we are entirely indebted to the Cherokee Indians. According to Dr. Garden, the discovery was made by them about forty years previous to the time he wrote (1764.) It soon became known to the white inhabitants, and in a short time was used extensively in Charlestown and throughout Carolina. Besides Dr. Garden, Drs. Lining* and Chalmers give accounts of its efficacy and general use at the time. It is needless to say that it retains to this day the high reputation which it acquired eighty years ago. In connection with the early history of the Pink root before the properties of it were precisely understood, Dr. Chalmers records the case of two healthy children both in one family, one of seven and the other of five years of age, who died on the same day, from convulsions induced by its use.†

Virginia could also boast of some distinguished men in the profession; and among these especially were *Clayton* and *Mitchell.* Dr. *John Clayton* was of English origin, and came to Virginia about the year 1705.‡ He was particularly eminent as a botanist, and devoted a long life to the investigations of the plants of Virginia. As the result of his labors, he published in 1743 a *Flora Virginica.* It was afterwards republished by Gronovius at Leyden, in 1762.§ Besides this,

* Of the anthelmintic virtues of the Indian Pink, being part of a letter from Dr. JOHN LINING, physician at Charlestown in South Carolina, to Dr. ROBERT WHYTT, Prof. of Medicine in the University of Edinburgh. Edinburgh Essays and observations, &c., vol. 1, p. 436. An account of the weather and diseases of South Carolina. Vol. 1, p. 66.

† On the weather and diseases of South Carolina. Vol. 1, p. 67.

‡ Thacher's Med. Biography, p. 224.

§ Flora Virginica exhibens plantas quas nobilissimus vir D. D. Johannes Claytonus, Med. Doct. &c., in Virginia crescentes observavit, collegit et obtuht D. Joh. Fred. Gronovio, cujus studio et opera descriptae et in ordinem sexualem systematicum redactae sistuntur. Lugduni Batavorum 1762.

he published in the Philosophical Transactions several papers in relation to the culture of the different varieties of tobacco, together with a full account of the medicinal plants of Virginia. The celebrated author of the Notes on Virginia, has left the following respectful testimony to the character of this eminent naturalist and physician: "This accurate observer was a native [incorrect] and resident of Virginia, passed a long life in exploring and describing its plants, and is supposed to have enlarged the botanical catalogue as much as almost any man who has lived."*

Dr. *John Mitchell* was another Englishman who emigrated to Virginia about the beginning of the last century, and no less distinguished for his attainments in medicine and natural history. The productions by which his name has been handed down to posterity are, "An Essay on the causes of the different colors of people in different climates," and "Letters on the yellow fever of Virginia." The first of these is a production of no ordinary character. It was published in the Philosophical Transactions of 1743, and occupies about fifty pages. The first part of this paper is occupied with the consideration of the cause of the color of the skin generally, and he endeavors to establish the following propositions: 1. That the color of white people proceeds from the color which the epidermis transmits; that is, from the color of the parts under the epidermis, rather than from any color of its own: 2. That the skins of negroes are of a thicker substance and denser texture than those of white people, and transmit no color through them: 3. That the part of the skin which appears black in negroes, is the corpus reticulare cutis, and external lamella of the epidermis; and all the other parts are of the same color in them with those

* Notes on Virginia, by Thomas Jefferson, p. 63.

of white people, except the fibres which pass between these
two parts: 4. That the color of negroes does not proceed
from any black humors or fluid parts contained in their
skins, for there is none such in any part of their bodies, more
than in white people: 5. The epidermis, especially its external lamella, is divided into two parts by its pores and
scales, two hundred times less than the particles of bodies,
on which their colors depend. Having established these propositions by a series of facts and reasonings, he comes to the
conclusion that the proximate cause of the color of negroes
is three-fold, viz: the opacity of their skins, proceeding
from the thickness and density of their texture, which obstructs the transmission of the rays of light from the white
and red parts below them; together with their greater re-
fractive power which absorbs those rays, and the smallness
of the particles of their skins, which hinder them from re-
flecting any light. The difference thus depending upon a
difference in the texture of the skins, he next proceeds to
show that the different colors of the human race can
readily be explained by the effect of climate and the mode
of life, in modifying the texture of the skin. He supports the
scriptural doctrine of the common origin of man, and
thinks the primitive color was a medium between white and
black, "from which primitive color the Europeans degen-
erated as much on the one hand as the Africans did on the
other; the Asiatics, unless, perhaps, where mixed with the
whiter Europeans, with most of the Americans, retaining the
primitive and original complexion."* Such is a brief account of this most ingenious and elaborate paper. Any analysis of it, however, must do it injustice. To appreciate the

* See the Abridgment of the Philosophical Transactions, by Drs.
Hutton, Shaw and Pearson, vol. 9, p. 50.

philosophical acumen and learning which it displays, it ought to be read at full length.

Another paper by Dr. Mitchell is an account of the yellow fever which prevailed in Virginia in 1741, of which I have already had occasion to speak in a previous part of this discourse. This was not published at the time, but the manuscript fell into the hands of Dr. Franklin, by whom, a short time before his death, it was given to Dr. Rush. It has since been published in Coxe's Medical Museum, and in the Medical and Philosophical Register of New York.†

Another physician of Virginia, and a native, Dr. *John Tennent*, deserves to be mentioned, as having written the first account of that valuable medicine, the *Polygala Seneka*. He appears to have been a connection of the celebrated Dr. Richard Mead, of London, and it was to him, that he communicated the first information on this subject.‡ The account which he gives is not without its interest. It seems that the plant had long been used by the Seneca tribe of Indians as a specific in cases of poisoning by the bite of a rattlesnake. They had inferred this from a supposed resemblance between the root of the plant and the rattle of the snake. Dr. Tennent had seen cases of this kind successfully treated by it, and from the analogy in the symptoms and those of peripneumony and pleurisy, he was led to try it in those diseases, and, as he relates, with great success. When the disease was of the acute inflammatory character he practised blood-letting. When it was of the nervous or bastard kind, or of long standing, he discarded not merely blood-letting,

† Two letters, vol. 4, pp. 183, 383.

‡ An Epistle to *Dr. Mead* concerning the Seneca Rattle-snake Root, by JOHN TENNENT. 8vo. Edinburgh, 1738. See Edinburgh Medical Essays and Observations, vol. 6, page 376.

but blisters and all other remedies, and trusted exclusively
to the snake-root, which he affirmed "scarce ever failed to
make a cure, and that in some desperate cases." He also
recommends it in rheumatism, dropsy and gout. He used it
both in powder and decoction—the latter however, he pre-
ferred. This was prepared by boiling 3 iij. of the bruised
root in a quart of water to near the half. Of this three spoons-
ful were given every six hours. Of the powder the dose was
35 grs. The effects, he says, are diuretic, diaphoretic,
cathartic, and sometimes emetic. The virtues of the polygala
had no sooner been promulgated in Europe, than they
were tested and confirmed by Bouvart and several other
French physicians. It is worthy of remark, that although
the efficiency of it against the bite of the rattlesnake has
proved fanciful, yet its reputation as a valuable adjuvant in
certain forms of pulmonary disease has been retained to the
present day. For the subsequent application of it too, as a
remedy in croup, we are indebted to an American physician,
Dr. *Archer,* of Maryland. By him it was originally recommended in this disease in the year 1806. To American
physicians, are we thus indebted for almost all our knowledge of this valuable plant.

Among the medical men of Pennsylvania, there are several who are entitled to notice, as having contributed to
the colonial literature of our profession. In 1740, Dr.
Thomas Cadwallader, of Philadelphia, published "An Essay on the Illiac Passion," in which he exposes the absurdity
of the practice then in vogue, viz: that of treating it by
quicksilver and drastic purges. He recommends in their
stead, mild cathartics, with the occasional use of opiates.‡
By Dr. *Thomas Bond,* an eminent physician of Philadelphia,

‡ Miller's Retrospect of the Eighteenth Century, vol. i. p. 317.

two communications were published in the London Medical Observations and Inquiries, one an account of a worm bred in the liver,§ 1754; another on the use of bark in scrofulous cases, 1759.|| The men, however, who were particularly distinguished, in Philadelphia, for their zeal in the cause of medical science, were Drs. *John Morgan* and *William Shippen,* both natives of that place, and the founders of the first medical school established in this country. Dr. Morgan, after studying medicine at home, went to Edinburgh, where he received the doctor's degree, on which occasion he published an elaborate thesis on the formation of pus—"Tentamen Medicum de Puris Confectione, Edinburgh, 1763." In this dissertation he maintained the doctrine that *pus is a secretion,* prepared by a peculiar action of the secretory vessels of the part. The credit of originality, as it regards this doctrine, has generally been awarded to the celebrated John Hunter. The evidence, however, appears to be conclusive, that he was anticipated by Dr. Morgan.* After receiving his degree at Edinburgh, he travelled for some time on the continent, industriously engaged in acquiring knowledge, and everywhere received with the highest honor. As a proof of the estimation in which he was held

§ Vol. 1, p. 68.
|| Vol. 2, p. 265.
* See Cullen's First Lines, edited by Prof. Charles Caldwell, vol. i. p. 225, note by Prof. Caldwell. Dr. James Curry, lecturer at Guy's Hospital, also gives the credit of priority to Dr. Morgan, and he adds: "I could not avoid giving that merit to Dr. Morgan, who discussed the question with great ingenuity, in his Inaugural Dissertation, on taking his degree at Edinburgh in 1763; whilst I could find no proof that Mr. Hunter had taught, or even adopted such an opinion, until a considerably later period." See London Med. and Phys. Journal for 1817; also, New England Journal of Med. and Surg., vol. vi., p. 404.

abroad, it is only necessary to state, that on his return home, in 1765, he was a fellow of the Royal Society of London, corresponding member of the Royal Academy of Surgery of Paris, and licentiate of the Royal Colleges of Physicians of London and Edinburgh. Notwithstanding his devotion to science, Dr. Morgan was not a prolific author. Besides his Thesis, all that we have left is his "Discourse," already noticed, "On the Institution of Medical Schools in America," in 1765, and "A Recommendation of Inoculation, According to Baron Dimsdale's Method," 1776.

Dr. Shippen was born in 1736, and about the year 1760 took his degree at Edinburgh, on which occasion he wrote and published a thesis, "De Placentae Cum Utero Nexu." Besides this I do not know that he published anything, but he is greatly and justly celebrated as the first professor of anatomy in this country.†

Last, though not least, the contributions of the eminent men who adorned our profession in *New York* require to be briefly commemorated. Among these, the first place is unquestionably due to *Cadwallader Colden*. He was a native of Scotland, and received his education at the university of Edinburgh. In 1718, he settled in New York. He soon, however, relinquished the practice of physic, and became a public character holding in succession the offices of sur-

† This was in 1765. A few years before this, anatomical lectures were delivered (that is, in the years 1754-5-6) at Newport, Rhode Island by *William Hunter,* M. D. Dr. Hunter was born in Scotland and was a relative of the celebrated Drs. Wm. and John Hunter. He was a graduate of the University of Edinburgh. He came to Rhode Island in the year 1752. According to Dr. Thacher, "advertisements of this Lecture may be seen in the Boston papers of that day." His manuscript Lectures are said to be still in existence. *See Thacher.*

veyor general of the province, member of the council, and finally lieutenant governor. Although thus withdrawn from the profession, he did not lose his fondness for medical and philosophical pursuits.

Among his medical productions is an "Account of the Climate and diseases of New York." This was published when he was surveyor general of the province, about the year 1720. It is an exceedingly interesting paper, giving as it does the only account we have of the climate and diseases of this city, at so early a period. In relation to consumption, now so fatally prevalent, he makes the following interesting remarks: "the air of the country being almost always clear, and its spring strong, we have few consumptions, or diseases of the lungs. People inclined to be consumptive in England, are often perfectly cured by our fine air, but if there be ulcers formed, they die in a little time."* He concludes his paper by saying that "the climate grows every day better as the country is cleared of the woods, and more healthy, as all the people that have long lived here testify. This has even been sensible to me, though I have been but twelve years in the country. I therefore doubt not but it will in time become one of the most agreeable and healthy climates on the face of the earth. As it is at present, I prefer it to the climate of England, and I believe most people that have lived any considerable time here, and are returned to England, will confirm this."† He also wrote, "observations on the Fever which prevailed in the city of New York in 1741-2," in which he made a number of valuable suggestions in relation to draining and purification, with the view of preventing

* Medical and Philosophical Register of New York, vol. i. p. 310.
† Medical and Philosophical Register of New York, vol. i. p. 310.

the recurrence of the disease.‡ For this the corporation of
the city presented him their thanks, and a plan for draining and cleaning the city was established, which was attended with the most salutary effects." Besides these, he
published a treatise "On the cure of cancer;" and another
"on the virtues of the great water dock," which is said to
have "introduced him to an acquaintance with Linnaeus.
In 1753 he addressed a letter to Dr. Fothergill of London,
giving an account of the *throat distemper,* which had been
previously described by Dr. Douglass. This was published
in the London Medical Observations and Enquiries.* In
this letter he gives a brief account of the progress of the disease after its first appearance at Kingston, in New Hamp-
shire in the year 1735. From thence he says "it spread west-
ward, but so gradually, that nearly two years elapsed before
it reached the Hudson river where Dr. Colden resided. For
some time it continued on the east side of the river; it then
passed to the west and made its appearance first in those
places to which the people of New England chiefly resorted
for trade, and in places through which they travelled. From
thence it continued to proceed westerly, till finally it spread
all over the British colonies. He then proceeds to give an
account of the symptoms and treatment of the disease, which
is chiefly interesting as confirming the account previously
given of it by Dr. Douglass of Boston. He acknowledges his
indebtedness to him in the following terms. "What I chiefly
learned, was from the late Dr. Douglass of Boston, a gentle-
man of great skill in medicine, and an accurate observer,
having corresponded with him while this distemper was
frequent in the part of the country where I lived."†

‡ Ib. vol. i, p. 324.
* Vol. i. p. 211.
† Medical Observations and Enquiries of London, vol. i. 211.

Although Dr. Colden has thus left several interesting papers on medical subjects, his principal attention was directed to scientific and literary pursuits. Botany was a favorite study. He described between three and four hundred plants, which were afterwards printed in the Acta Upsaliensa. In honor of his daughter, who imbibed the ardor of her parent in this science, Linnaeus named a plant of the tetrandrous class, that was first described by her, *Coldenia*. His "history of the Five Indian Nations," is a work of high interest and value, even at the present day.‡ He also published a work on the cause of gravitation. This was afterwards enlarged and republished in 1751, by Dodsley, in 1 vol. 4to., entitled, "The principles of action in Motion."

Altogether the name of Colden is one of the most distinguished in our colonial annals. He corresponded with the most distinguished men abroad, as well as those in this country and especially with Dr. Franklin. They appear to have been men of similar tastes and sympathies, and interchanged opinions continually on electricity, philosophy and other scientific subjects. Dr. Colden also first suggested the establishment of the American Philosophical Society. As a proof of the ingenuity and versatility of his genius, it is worthy of record that Dr. Colden suggested in a letter to Dr. Franklin, in 1743, a new method of printing, which is now commonly known as *Stereotyping*.* This letter is published in

‡ History of the Five Indian Nations of Canada, 8vo. London 1747.

* In some comments upon this letter the editors of the Register make the following remarks. "The mode of printing above described is now known by the term *Stereotype*, and it is a curious fact that the stereotype process, said to have been invented by M. Herhan in Paris, and now practiced by him in that city, under let-

full, together with the answer of Dr. Franklin, in the American Medical and Philosophical Register, vol. 1, p. 439.

Dr. *John Bard* was long an eminent practitioner of New York. His professional writings, however, are few. They are —"A case of extra Uterine Foetus," published in 1760, in the London Obs. and Inq's.;† several papers on the nature and character of the yellow fever, and "An essay on the nature and cause of the malignant pleurisy;" which proved so fatal to the inhabitants of Huntington and some other places in Long Island in the winter of 1749.‡

Of the physicians of New York, none were more distinguished for their learning and ability, than Dr. *Peter Middleton.* On the formation of the medical school of New York, he was appointed professor of the theory of physic. At the opening of the school, in 1767, he delivered a discourse in which he took an extensive survey of the state of medicine among the different nations of the globe. This production was afterwards published, and affords ample proof of the

ters patent of Napoleon is precisely the same as that spoken of by Dr. Colden, more than sixty years ago. It is more than probable that when Dr. Franklin went to France, he communicated Dr. Colden's "new method of printing," to some artists there, and that it lay dormant until about sixteen years since; when Herhan, a German who had been an assisant to M. Didot, the printer and type founder of Paris, but then separated from him, took it up in opposition to M. Didot. We have conversed with gentlemen who have seen M. Herhan's method of stereotyping, and they describe it to be exactly what Governor Colden invented. This fact established, there can be no doubt that M. Herhan is indebted to America for the celebrity he has obtained in France." American Med. and Phil. Register, vol. 1, p. 443.

† Vol. ii. p. 369.

‡ Med. and Philos. Register, vol. i. p. 409.

learning and ability of the author.* He also wrote a valuable practical letter on the "Croup," already alluded to."†

Dr. *John Jones* was a native of Jamaica, Long-Island, and was born in 1729. Having acquired the elements of his profession at home, he repaired to Europe, and enjoyed the advantages of tuition under the most renowned men of our profession at London, Leyden, Paris and Edinburgh. In 1751, he received the degree of Doctor of Medicine at the University of Rheims. On his return to his native country, he established himself in the city of New York, and speedily rose to the highest eminence. Although educated in every department of his profession, yet he devoted himself specially to surgery. He was the first surgeon who performed the operation of lithotomy in New York, and with so much skill and success that he not merely established the safety of the operation, but was extensively employed to perform it.‡ In 1761, he was selected to fill the honorable station of

* A Medical discourse or an historical inquiry into the ancient and present state of medicine; the substance of which was delivered at the opening of the medical school in the city of New York: by Peter Middleton, M.D., and Prof. of the theory of physic in King's College: New York, 1769, pp. 72. A copy of this is in possession of the writer.

† This letter was published in 1780, and addressed to Dr. Richard Bayley. In it, he sanctions the practice of Dr. Bayley, as confirmed by his own experience. See New York Med. Repository, vol. xiv. p. 347.

‡ Dr. Mease, in his interesting Memoir of Dr. Jones, states that "this operation had been frequently attempted in other States, but the want of success attending it, was generally so great, as to prevent it from being performed in future. The fortunate manner, however, in which those cases under his (Dr. Jones') care succeeded, fully proved it was no longer the dangerous operation many had been made to apprehend, an opinion which induced them rather to submit to a miserable life, than to suffer the risk of falling a sacrifice to the means instituted for their relief." American Med. and Phil. Register, vol. 4, p. 328.

Professor of Surgery in the Medical School of New York. This was the first regular professorship of surgery established in this country, and Dr. Jones was eminently qualified to fill it. He was not a mere mechanical surgeon, and he was well fitted by education and his various accomplishments to become the instructor of others. The only work he has left us is a volume upon wounds and fractures, which was first published in 1776.§ In the situation in which the colonies were then placed, this was a most acceptable present, both to the profession and to the public. It was so well received, that a second edition was called for the same year. Although a plain and unpretending work, it was admirably fitted to the purposes for which it was intended, and it shows the author to have been a man of the strong sense, combined with a thorough knowledge of his subject. The motive which prompted him to this undertaking, is thus expressed in his dedication: "To Doctor Thomas Cadwallader, Physician, in Philadelphia."

"The present calamitous situation of this country, in a peculiar manner demands the aid and assistance of every virtuous citizen; and though few men are possessed of those superior talents which are requisite to heal such mighty evils as now threaten the whole body politic with ruin and desolation; yet, every man has it in his power to contribute something to so desirable an end; and if he cannot cure the fatal diseases of his country, it will at least afford him some consolation, to have poured a little balm into her bleeding wounds." p. 3.

§ Plain Concise Practical Remarks on the Treatment of Wounds and Fractures; to which is added an Appendix on Camp and Military Hospitals. Principally designed for the use of young military and naval surgeons in North America; by John Jones, M.D., professor of surgery in King's College, New York, p. 114—Philadelphia, 1776.

The introduction to the work, addressed "to the students, and young practitioners of surgery, through all America," abounds in just sentiments, eminently valuable at the time they were published, and not unworthy of recollection at the present day. His ideas of the qualifications necessary to make a really good surgeon were by no means low. "The proper requisites of this respectable character," says he, "are only to be found in a liberal education, furnishing every means of acquiring that knowledge, which must be ripened by experience, and graced by the constant practice of attention, tenderness and humanity. A judicious surgeon will always find his powers and abilities of assisting the wretched proportionable to the time he has spent, and the pains he has bestowed in acquiring the proper knowledge of his profession," p. 6. He deprecates the separation of physic from surgery as injurious to both. "In most European countries," says he, 'an invidious distinction has prevailed between physic and surgery, but in this part of the world the two professions are generally united; indeed both the branches of medicine are in the very nature of things, so intimately connected, as not to admit of absolute separation without manifest inquiry to each," p. 9. He concludes with the following remarks: "Surgery may, with great propriety, be divided into medical and manual;—the first comprehends an infinite variety of diseases, which require the assistance of both internal and external applications;—the last is confined to those cases which admit of relief from the hand alone, or assisted with instruments.

Hence it will appear very evident how necessary it is for the student in surgery to make himself thoroughly acquainted with most of those branches of medicine which are requisite to form an accomplished physician.

Besides a competent acquaintance with the learned languages, which are to lay the foundation of every other acquisition; he must possess an accurate knowledge of the structure of the human body, acquired not only by attending anatomical lectures, but by frequent dissections of dead bodies with his own hands. This practice cannot be too warmly recommended to students in surgery. It is from this source and a knowledge in hydraulics, they must derive any adequate notions of the animal economy or physiology. Chemistry and Materia Medica are very necessary to a right understanding of pharmacy or composition. To these should be added some progress in the mathematics and mechanics, which I will venture to assert, may be applied with much more utility and safety to the science of surgery than physic. But there must be a happiness, as well as art, to complete the character of the great surgeon.

He ought to have firm steady hands, and be able to use both alike; a strong clear sight, and above all a mind calm and intrepid, yet humane and compassionate, avoiding every appearance of horror and cruelty to his patient, amid the most severe operations." p. 9, 10, 11.

From the foregoing it appears that Dr. Jones considered a liberal preliminary education "essential to form the good surgeon as well as the good physician," and the whole extract is exceedingly interesting, not merely as an evidence of the liberal views of the author, but as showing the high standard of professional excellence which was beginning to be enforced at that early day. The only other production on record of Dr. Jones is an interesting paper on "Anthrax," in the first part of volume 1, of the Transactions of the College of Physicians of Philadelphia.

Altogether, Dr. Jones has left behind him a most enviable reputation. He was the physician of Washington and

Franklin, the latter of whom he attended in his last illness.*
Not merely as the skilful operator, but as the scientific surgeon, and the first teacher of surgery in the colonies, he
justly deserves to be styled the *father of American surgery*.

Among the medical men of New York who commenced
their career before the revolution, Dr. *Samuel Bard* is not
the least deserving of notice. Dr. Bard was born in 1742, and
after having received a liberal education at King's (now
Columbia) College, together with some preliminary instruction in medicine from his father, Dr. John Bard, he set sail
for Europe in 1760, where he prosecuted his professional
studies, partly in London, but principally in Edinburgh,
where, after remaining three years, he graduated in 1765.
While a student at Edinburgh, he distinguished himself
as a botanist, and obtained the prize offered by Dr. Hope,

* The following interesting account of the last moments of
Franklin, written by Dr. Jones, was published at the time: "The
stone, with which he had been afflicted for several years, had for the
last twelve months of his life confined him chiefly to his bed; and
during the extremely painful paroxysms, he was obliged to take
large doses of laudanum to mitigate his tortures; still, in the inter-
vals of pain, he not only amused himself by reading and conversing
cheerfully with his family and a few friends who visited him, but
was often employed in doing business of a public as well as of a private nature, with various persons who waited upon him for that purpose; and in every instance displayed not only the readiness and
disposition to do good, which were the distinguished characteristics
of his life, but the fullest and clearest possession of his uncommon
abilities. He also not unfrequently indulged in those jeux d'esprit,
and entertaining anecdotes, which were the delight of all who heard
him.

"About sixteen days before his death, he was seized with a fever-
ish disposition, without any particular symptoms attending it till
the third or fourth day, when he complained of a pain in the left
breast, which increased till it became extremely acute, attended by

professor of botany in the University of Edinburgh, for the best herbarium of indigenous plants growing within ten miles of Edinburgh.* On the occasion of his graduation he published an Inaugural Thesis on opium, in the latin language.† This is no mean production. Considering the period when this essay appeared, the age of the writer, and the manner in which the investigation with regard to the effects of opium was conducted, it shows the author to have been endowed with no ordinary powers. It attracted the notice of the celebrated Haller, and is also mentioned by Crumpe, in his valuable work on opium, with high com-

a cough and laborious breathing. During this state, when the severity of his pains drew forth a groan of complaint, he would observe that he was afraid he did not bear them as he ought; acknowledging his grateful sense of the many blessings he had received from the Supreme Being, who had raised him from small and low beginnings, to such high rank and consideration among men; and had no doubt but that his present afflictions were kindly intended to wean him from a world in which he was no longer fit to act the part assigned him. In this frame of body and mind he continued until five days before his death, when the pain and difficulty of breathing entirely left him, and his family were flattering themselves with the hopes of his recovery; but an imposthume which had formed in his lungs, suddenly burst, and discharged a quantity of matter which he continued to throw up while he had power, but as that failed, the organs of respiration became gradually oppressed; a calm lethargic state succeeded, and on the 17th day of April, 1790, about eleven o'clock at night, he quietly expired, closing a long and useful life of eighty-four years and three months." Mease's Memoir.

* This collection is yet in existence; at least it was so a few years since. Dr. Mitchill states that one of the volumes was in his possession containing about one hundred plants; and after the lapse of fifty years was in good preservation. It was lettered, *E Plantis circa Edinam natis.*—Mitchill's Discourse, p. 13.

† Tentamen Medicum Inaugurale, de viribus Opii. Edin. 1765. pp. 49.

mendation. At the period when Dr. Bard studied, the subject of opium was not so well understood as it is at present, and a great difference of opinion existed in relation to several points which Dr. Bard undertook to investigate. These were, the part of the system upon which opium primarily operated; whether its effects on the pulse were stimulant or sedative, and whether it increased or diminished animal heat. Dr. Bard contended that it acted primarily on the nervous system and not on the blood; that its action was uniformly sedative on the pulse, and that it lessened animal heat. With regard to the pulse, he performed a number of experiments upon himself as well as some of his friends, confirmatory of this opinion. The general conclusions to which he came in relation to the virtues of opium were the following: 1. That it produces hilarity of mind; 2. That it retards the action of the heart and arteries, and renders the pulse fuller; 3. That it diminishes animal heat; 4. That it lessens all the secretions with the exception of the perspiration, which it increases; 5. That it constipates the bowels; 6. That it sometimes suppresses the urine; 7. That it renders respiration slower; 8. That it causes a sense of fullness and stricture about the head and chest; 9. That it lessens pain, resolves spasms, recruits the body exhausted by labor, causes sleep, and sometimes produces itching of the skin.

After his graduation, he returned to New York in his twenty-fourth year, and according to Dr. Mitchill, might be "considered as the most accomplished young physician that New York could then boast."*

Dr. Bard had scarcely settled himself in New York, before we find him engaged in two enterprises of great interest, both to the profession and the public—and these were the

* A Discourse on the Life and Character of Samuel Bard, M. D., &c., by SAMUEL S. MITCHILL, M.D., LL.D., p. 17.

organization of a medical faculty and the establishment of
a public hospital. In 1767, the Trustees of King's College
established a medical faculty, and it is an unequivocal proof
of the high estimation in which Dr. Bard was held, when
we find him appointed to one of the most important chairs,
that of the Practice of Medicine, and more particularly so,
when we find the men associated with him were not only
much more advanced in years, but men of high professional
standing. In this capacity Dr. Bard soon distinguished himself by an introductory which he delivered at the commencement in 1768, in which he advocated with so much zeal the
necessity of a public hospital, that it led at once to the establishment of that noble institution, the *New York Hospital.*

In 1771, Dr. Bard published an essay† on the sore-throat
distemper, which was then prevalent in New York, and
which attracted much professional as well as general interest.
This essay was first published in the Transactions of the
American Philosophical Society, and communicated to John
Morgan, M.D., F.R.S. Vol. 1, p. 388.

This is the least satisfactory of all the productions of Dr.
Bard. The late Dr. Mitchill says of it, "the disease he describes has puzzled the physicians who have read his publication. For Cullen, the acute nosologist, places it in the list
of works on the cynanche maligna; while Albers, the successful competitor for the Buonopartean medal, quotes it as
a treatise on cynanche trachealis. The former classes it with
the writings on the malignant or ulcerous sore throat, while

† "An Enquiry into the nature, cause and cure of the Angina
Suffocativa, or sore-throat distemper, as it is commonly called, by
the inhabitants of this city and colony." By SAMUEL BARD, M.D., and
Professor of the Practice of Physic, in Kings College, New York. Is
certe curraturus quem prima origo causae non fefellerit. Celsus.
New York, 1771. Dedicated to Cad. Colden, Lieut. Gov. of the
Province, page 33.

the latter ranks it with the publications on croup or trachealis infantum."* The truth is, that at the time Dr.
Bard wrote, no accurate discrimination was made between the two
diseases, and as both the sore-throat disease and the croup
prevailed at this time in New York, it was not singular that
they were generally confounded with each other. Dr. Bard
fell into the common mistake on this subject, as is apparent
from his essay. He says, "I am led to conclude that the disease called by the Italians *Morbus Strangulatorius,* the
Croup of Dr. Home, the *sore-throat* of Huxham and Fothergill, this *disease* and *that* described by Dr. Douglass, of Boston, however they may differ in the symptoms of putrescency
and malignancy, do all bear an essential affinity and relation
to each other—are apt to run into one another, and in fact
arise from the same fever," &c. page 19. In his essay, accordingly, Dr. Bard mentions symptoms peculiar to both diseases; and also recommends a treatment fully suited to the
one and partly to the other.

The remainder of the history of Dr. Bard's life belongs
to a period not embraced in the present sketch. In 1811 he
was appointed President of the College of Physicians and
Surgeons of New York, a place he filled with grace and
dignity. He also published a work on *obstetrics,* with several other minor productions. Finally, in 1821, at the age
of seventy-nine, he closed his useful life, full of years and
full of honor, with the dignified composure and the firm
hope of a christian.

Before closing this account of our colonial medical literature, it would be unjust not to notice the Transactions
of a Society, which contributed in no small degree to raise

* A Discourse on the Life and Character of Samuel Bard, M.D.,
LL.D., &c., by SAMUEL L. MITCHILL, M.D., &c., p. 21: New York,
1821.

the scientific character of the country. I mean, the American Philosophical Society.† The first volume of their proceedings was published anterior to the revolution, (1771) and contains some papers on important medical subjects. It may be stated, too, that four American physicians were elected fellows of the Royal Society of London, before the revolution. These were Drs. Boylston, Mitchill (of Virginia) , Garden, and Morgan. Besides these there were ten other Americans who had been raised to the same honor, viz: four of the name of Winthrop, Paul Dudley, President Leverett, Thomas Brattle, Cotton Mather, Benjamin Franklin, and David Rittenhouse.*

No medical journal of any description appears to have been published until after the war of our independence, and the only inagural dissertation that was published was from the New York college in 1771, by Samuel Kissam, M.D., on the Anthelmintic Virtue of the *Phaseolus Zuratensis Siliqua Hirsuta,* or Cow-Itch, a copy of which may be seen in the library of the New York Historical Society.

† This Society was organized in the year 1744. An interesting letter from Dr. Franklin to Dr. Colden, dated April 5, 1774, gives an account of the original members comprising the Society. They were the following, viz: Dr. Thomas Bond as physician, Mr. John Bartram as botanist, Mr. Thomas Godfrey as mathematician, Mr. Samuel Rhodes as mechanician, Mr. William Parsons as Geographer, Dr. Phineas Bond as general natural philosopher, Mr. Thomas Hopkinson, President, Mr. William Coleman, Treasurer, Benjamin Franklin, Secretary. *See American Medical and Philosophical Register,* vol. ii. p. 203, for the letter itself as well as a facsimile.

* Ramsay's America, vol. i. p. 271.

Chapter Four

MEDICAL EDUCATION AND
INSTITUTIONS

U NDER THIS HEAD MAY BE EMBRACED ALL THOSE ACTS
and establishments of the colonial governments,
whose object was the preservation of the public
health, as well as those institutions of a public nature, which
originated from the combination of individual enterprise
and liberality.

From the commercial character of the country, it may
readily be supposed, that our first medical establishments
were lazarettos, or hospitals intended for the reception of
seamen and others infected with contagious disorders. Accordingly we find a hospital of this description established
by Massachusetts, nearly one hundred and fifty years ago,
at Rainsford island, in the harbor of Boston. Another was at
an early period erected on State island in the Delaware, and
appropriated to similar purposes for the port of Philadelphia. After the practice of inoculation had become settled,
hospitals were gradually established in different parts of the
country, for the purpose of carrying patients through this
process. Several of this description were in existence shortly
after the middle of the last century. These were, however,
entirely the result of private enterprise, without any legis-
lative aid, and were therefore, only of temporary duration.
Among the physicians who devoted themselves to this kind
of business, Dr. Barnet of New Jersey seems to have been

the most conspicuous. So common had these establishments become, that laws in relation to them were passed by the authorities in several of the colonies.*

Useful as the foregoing institutions undoubtedly were, they could not have produced any effect of consequence upon the existing state of medical science. In 1750, a project of a higher order was set on foot in Philadelphia; this was the establishment of a hospital, upon the plan and embracing all the advantages of the European hospitals, and the individual with whom it originated was Dr. Thomas Bond. No sooner was the object proposed to the citizens of Philadelphia, than measures were adopted to carry it into execution. For that purpose, a petition was presented to the Assembly of the colony soliciting the aid of that body, the result of which was a grant of £2000, on condition that an equal sum should be raised by subscription. The proposed amount was speedily raised; and early in the year 1752, patients were admitted into a building which had been procured for their temporary accommodation. The erection of the present building was not commenced until 1755. In the year 1769, a similar project was started in New York, and the credit of first suggesting it is due to the late *Dr. Samuel Bard*. In consequence of a public discourse delivered by him, a general interest was excited in the measure.† The

* See appendix E.

† The agency of Dr. Bard is mentioned in the following terms by Dr. Middleton, in his discourse delivered 1769. "The necessity and usefulness of a public infirmary, has been so warmly and pathetically set forth in a discourse delivered by Dr. Samuel Bard, at the commencement in May last, that his Excellency Sir Henry Moore immediately set on foot a subscription for that purpose, to which himself and most of the gentlemen present liberally contributed. His Excellency also recommended it, in the most pressing manner, to the Assembly of the province, as an object worthy of

liberal contributions of the governor of the province, (Sir Henry Moore,) the corporation of the city, and the legislature of the province, enabled the governors to commence the erection of the building in 1773. After being nearly completed, it accidentally took fire, and was nearly consumed, in 1775. The present building was not completed until 1791, when it was opened for the reception of patients.* These were all the hospitals that were attempted anterior to the revolution.

Among the most singular features connected with the history of our colonial medicine, is the fact that so little attention was paid to professional education. This is the more remarkable, inasmuch as our colonial ancestors were fully alive to the importance of general instruction, and the most honorable efforts were made to establish it on a respectable foundation. So early as the year 1638, Harvard University, in Massachusetts, was founded. In 1691, William and Mary College, in Virginia; in 1700, Yale College, in Connecticut; and in 1746, Princeton College, in New Jersey, were severally established; yet in none of them was any provision made for instruction in medical science. With the single exception, too, of New York, already noticed, and that so late as 1760, the law imposed no qualifications upon those who entered the profession, nor were they subjected to

their attention; and the corporation of the city have given assurance of granting a very valuable and commodious lot of ground for erecting the building upon; so that there is now almost a certain prospect of this benevolent and humane foundation soon taking place; and as it is to be on the most catholic and unexceptionable plan, it is to be hoped that it will meet with the countenance and encouragement of every compassionate and good member of society, whatever party or denomination he may choose to be distinguished by on other occasions." Note p. 60.

* An account of the New York Hospital, 1811.

any examinations. The education of physicians, therefore, at this period, restricted as it was to the personal instruction of those with whom they studied, must have been limited indeed. The only mode of supplying this deficiency, was by resorting to foreign countries; and it appears that almost all the distinguished physicians who flourished anterior to the revolution, had received their education in Europe. It is a fact certainly highly honorable and worthy of record, that Harvard College no sooner began to send forth her graduates, than some of them found their way to foreign universities, where they obtained the degree of doctor of medicine. In 1642, Samuel Bellingham graduated at the first commencement at Harvard, and shortly afterwards obtained a doctor's degree at Leyden. In 1650, John Glover and Leonard Hoar left the college, and were afterwards honored with the doctorate abroad, the former at Aberdeen, the latter at Cambridge in England. Hoar afterwards became president of Harvard college. In 1674, Edmund Davie graduated, and subsequently was made an M.D. at Padua.†
As may be supposed, this practice became more and more common, till the period of the revolution; and this, together with the number of foreign physicians of talent and education who emigrated to this country, tended, in no inconsiderable degree, to correct the deficiencies of domestic instruction. The first attempt at establishing a regular system of medical instruction in this country, was not made until a very few years before the revolution; and for this we are indebted to Drs. *William Shippen* and *John Morgan,* both natives of Pennsylvania, who projected the plan during the prosecution of their studies abroad. In 1762, Dr. Shippen returned to his native country, and in that year delivered a course of lectures of anatomy to a class of stu-

† See the catalogue of the graduates of Harvard College.

dents amounting to twelve in number. The lectures were repeated in 1763 and '64. In the following year Dr. Morgan, who had just returned from Europe, pronounced "A Discourse upon the Institution of Medical Schools in America," before the trustees of the college, in which he proposed a plan for teaching the different branches of medicine, and portrayed with prophetic ardor the blessings which would flow from such a measure. "Perhaps," said he, "this medical institution, the first of the kind in America, though small in its beginning, may receive a constant increase of strength and annually exert new vigor. It may collect a number of young persons, of more than ordinary abilities, and so improve their knowledge as to spread its reputation to distant parts. By sending them abroad duly qualified, or by exciting an emulation amongst men of parts and literature, it may give birth to other useful institutions of a similar nature, or occasional rise, by its example, to numerous societies of different kinds, calculated to spread the light of knowledge through the whole American continent, whereever inhabited." p. 58.

Happily he spoke to a body of men capable of entering into his expanded views; and measures were soon after adopted for forming a medical faculty. Dr. *Morgan* was appointed professor of the theory and practice of medicine, and Dr. *Shippen,* professor of anatomy and surgery. The other stations were not immediately filled. In 1768, Dr. *Adam Kuhn,** a pupil of Linnaeus, who had just returned

* Dr. Adam Kuhn was a native of Germantown, near Philadelphia, and born 1741. After receiving an elementary education in this country, he proceeded to Europe and for two years studied medicine at the University of Upsal, of which the celebrated Linnaeus was one of the professors. He appears to have been a favorite pupil of that great man. After spending another year in

to his native country, was chosen professor of botany and materia medica; and in 1769, Dr. *Rush,* who had just finished his education at Edinburgh, was chosen to the chemical chair. At the same time, Dr. *Thomas Bond* gave clinical lectures at the Pennsylvania hospital. Being thus provided with professors on the most important branches of medicine, the school went into complete operation, and the lectures were continued to the year 1775, when they were suspended by the war of the revolution. Dr. Shippen at this time had delivered fourteen courses, and the annual number of students had increased to between thirty and forty.*

New York soon became emulous of the example set her by Philadelphia, and in 1767 adopted measures for extending similar advantages to medical students. The scheme of a medical college was projected by a number of medical gentlemen, who were afterwards appointed professors. They submitted it to the trustees of King's, now Columbia College. By them it was promptly and cordially received, and the following professors unanimously appointed: *Samuel Clossey,* M.D.,† professor of anatomy; *John Jones,* M.D.,

London, he proceeded to Edinburgh, where he took his degree of doctor of Medicine, in 1767, on which occasion he published a *Thesis de Lavatione Frigida,* dedicated to Linnaeus. Dr. Kuhn was no author, but eminent as a practical physician and a useful teacher. He died at the age of 75, in the year 1817. *Eclectic Repertory,* vol. 8.

* Eulogium on Dr. William Shippen, by Caspar Wistar, M.D., p. 27, 1818.

† Dr. Clossey was an Irishman by birth, and a graduate of Trinity College, Dublin. Previously to his emigration to this country he had gained distinction at home, both as a practitioner and an author. He had published a valuable work entitled "Observations on some of the Diseases of the Human Body; chiefly taken from the Dissections of Morbid Bodies." 8vo. This appeared in London in 1763.

professor of surgery; *Peter Middleton*, M.D.,‡ professor of the theory of physic; *James Smith*, M.D.,§ professor of chemistry and materia medica; *John V. B. Tennent*, M.D.,* professor of midwifery, and *Samuel Bard*, M.D., professor of the practice of physic.

These gentlemen were fully competent to the enterprize they had undertaken. Their learning and abilities were unquestionable, and the manner in which they discharged their several duties seems to have been highly satisfactory. At the opening of the College, public introductories were delivered, which drew forth warm marks of approbation

As an evidence of his general attainments, is the fact of his being appointed, in 1765, professor of natural philosophy in King's College, now Columbia College, New York. The political difficulties in this country are said to have induced him to return to his native country, where he died a short time after his arrival.—See *Thacher's Medical Biography, Francis' Account of the College of Physicians and Surgeons of N.Y., Moore's Historical Sketch of Columbia College.*

‡ Of Dr. Middleton I have already spoken. I may add, that in 1750, in connection with Dr. J. Bard, he dissected a human body, and injected the blood vessels; the first attempt of the kind of which we have any record in this country. He died in the city of New York in 1781.

§ Dr. Smith was a brother of Wm. Smith, the historian of the State of New York. He received his medical education chiefly in Europe, and was graduated doctor of medicine at Leyden, on which occasion he defended an inaugural dissertation, "De Febre Intermittente." He is admitted by all to have been eminently learned, though too theoretical and fanciful, both as a practitioner of the healing art, and in his course of public instruction. He died at an advanced age, in the city of New York, in 1812.—*See Thacher's Med. Biography.*

* Dr. Tennent was a native of New Jersey, and had received the benefits of European medical education. He appears to have been an able lecturer. He died at an early age, in the West Indies, where he had gone for the benefit of his health.

from the trustees of the college. The following appears on
the minutes. At a meeting of the Governors, on the 25th of
November, 1767: it was "Ordered, that Mr. Attor'y General, the Reverend Mr. Auchmuty, and the Reverend Mr.
Cooper, be a committee to communicate to the several
medical professors, the high opinion this corporation enter-
tains of the learning and abilities whereby they have re-
spectively distinguished themselves, particularly in their
introductory lectures; to thank them for the zeal they have
expressed for the honor of this seminary, and the pains they
have taken to promote its interest, and to signify their
hopes that the said professors, by a continuance of their
services, will render the science of medicine much more
respectable than it hath hitherto been in this country, to
their own honor, the reputation of the college, and the
great emolument of the public."†

A measure so honorable to those immediately concerned
in effecting it, and to the city itself, promised not merely to
elevate the character of our profession, but to be productive
of general good to the community. The fair prospects thus
anticipated, were all arrested by the war.

The schools thus started in Philadelphia and New York,
were the only ones attempted before the revolution. The
first medical degrees were given by the college of New
York. In 1769, the degree of *Batchelor* in medicine was conferred upon Samuel Kissam and Robert Tucker. In 1770,
the degree of *Doctor* in medicine was conferred upon the
last of these gentlemen, and in May of the following year,
upon the former. In June, 1771, the degree of Doctor in
medicine was conferred on four students, by the Philadelphia college, being the first given by that institution.

†An Historical Sketch of Columbia College, in the City of New
York. By N. F. Moore. N. York: 1846. p. 53.

The establishment of Medical Faculties was unquestionably the most important event which had yet taken place in the history of our colonial medicine. It at once presented our profession in a new and imposing attitude before the public, and is associated with many circumstances of high interest. Not the least of these is, that it was the result entirely of *individual enterprise,* and originated in the bosom of the profession itself. The men who conceived it, too, were prepared to carry it through. The college in New York, especially, Minerva like, came into existence ready armed and equipped for the purposes of education in all the different branches of medical science. Although thus originating with individuals, the project was not premature or visionary—both the profession and the public were prepared for it, and it was no sooner started than it seems to have met with general favor.

There is another circumstance connected with the establishment of our first medical institutions which is deserving of especial notice, and that is the high value which at that early day was attached to *preliminary education.* On this subject Drs. Morgan and Middleton have left on record sentiments so creditable to themselves as men of cultivated minds, that I cannot refrain from quoting them.

"It will not be improper, however, to observe here that young men ought to come well prepared for the study of medicine, by having their minds enriched with all the aids they can receive from the languages, and the liberal arts. Latin and Greek are very necessary to be known by a physician. The latter contains the rich original treasures of ancient medical science and of the first parents of the healing art. The former contains all the wealth of more modern literature. It is the vehicle of knowledge in which the learned men of every nation in Europe choose to convey their sentiments, and communicate their discoveries to the world. As it is the best known of the dead languages, it is chosen as the most proper one, by the various nations of Europe, for a medium of intercourse among the learned, that is equally attainable by every one of them. Hence it becomes indispensably necessary for a physician, who is to derive his knowledge from so many different sources, to be well acquainted with Latin.

The French language has prevailed much in Europe. The advantages which we may reap from the writings of many eminent men, and of many learned societies which are published in French, make the knowledge of this language very valuable also to a physician. An acquaintance with mathematics and natural philosophy we cannot dispense with, since we can go but small lengths in natural or medical inquiries without their assistance. Happy are we to have all these taught in such perfection in this place. Destitute of that general knowledge which unveils to us the operations of nature, we cannot penetrate into those truths, that form the rules by which we ought to conduct ourselves in the cure of diseases.

There is no art yet known that may not contribute somewhat to the improvement of medicine; nor is there any one which requires more assistance than that of physic from every other science. Let young men, therefore, who would engage in the pursuit of Medicine, of Surgery, make use of all their industry to possess themselves in good time of these acquisitions. They are necessary to facilitate a progress in the healing arts; they embellish the understanding, and give many peculiar advantages, unattainable without them." Discourse p. 18, 19.

In the same spirit speaks Dr. Middleton: "No pupil ought to apply himself to the study of physic, till he has previously laid the foundation in a competent knowledge of classical learning, and some general acquaintance with the Mathematics and Natural Philosophy. No expense ought to be put in balance with the acquisition of every necessary branch of instruction, to insure a successful practice. He, who considers how he may go the cheapest way to work, too often purchases the name for the reality, the shadow for the substance. A candid and cursory view of the established practitioners here, and in the country around, will soon convince the most incredulous of the truth of this observation." p. 65.

It is mortifying to reflect that after the lapse of upwards of eighty years, the subject of preliminary education is precisely where it was. By enlightened individuals, the most glowing exhortations have been made from time to time in relation to its necessity and importance. As yet, however, no measure has been adopted by any of our colleges or public authorities to enforce this most radical of all reforms. Until this shall be done, it is needless to expect that our profession shall attain the elevation and dignity to which she is justly entitled.

With regard to the works that were commonly read and studied, the following is stated by Bartlett. "Though the works of Hippocrates, Galen, Stahl and others, were not unknown, those of Sydenham, and his followers, were principally studied by our oldest practitioners, till the time of Boerhaave, whose invaluable labors commenced in 1701, which, with the commentaries of Van Swieten; the practical writings of Whytt, Mead, Brooks and Huxham; the physiology of Haller; the anatomy of Cowper, Kiel, Douglass, Cheselden, Munro, and Winslow; the surgery of Heister, Sharp, Le Dran and Pott; the midwifery of Smellie and

Hunter; and the Materia Medica of Lewis, were in general use at our political separation from the British Empire.*

I have now completed the task which I proposed in the commencement of this discourse, which was to give a sketch of the state of medicine during our colonial existence. The revolutionary war succeeded. During that eventful period, our profession stood firm in their country's cause; and the names of Warren,† Mercer‡ and Rush,§ show that they were not idle spectators of the fray. Nothing was done, however, for the advancement of medical science. The newly formed medical colleges were broken up, and all the energies of the country directed to the attainment of a nation's highest hope and ambition. The revolution accomplished, and an independent government established, a new career was commenced. In common with everything else, medicine felt the sacred impulse, and during the brief period of our independence, how has the scene changed? Instead of the feeble

* A Dissertation on the progress of Medical Science in the Commonwealth of Massachusetts. By Josiah Bartlett. Communications of the Medical Society of Massachusetts, vol. 3, p. 240.

† Major General Joseph Warren was born at Roxbury near Boston, in 1741. He studied medicine and practised his profession at Boston. At the first breaking out of the revolution, he turned his attention to arms, and was slain at the battle of Bunker Hill, June 17, 1775. See Thacher's Medical Biography.

‡ "Hugh Mercer, M.D. a general in the revolutionary war, was a distinguished physician, who, like Warren, fell in the defence of the liberties of his country. He was a native of Scotland, and educated at Edinburgh. He early emigrated to Virginia, and settled at Fredericksburgh, where he practiced medicine for several years with great reputation. During the revolution, he zealously engaged in defence of the liberties of his adopted country, and fell in the battle of Princeton, 1777." Prof. Sewall's Lecture, 1825, p. 60.

§ Dr. Rush was a member of the Congress of 1775, and one of the signers of the declaration of independence.

beginnings of one or two institutions, twenty-eight well established medical colleges are now to be found in different parts of our country; every city has its hospitals; a thriving professional literature has sprung up among us, and we can now boast of authors whom we are not ashamed to mention along with those of European birth. What nation ever accomplished so much in an equal space of time, and under equal circumstances?

APPENDIX

(A)

AN ACT

To regulate the Practice of Physick and Surgery in the City of New York.

Passed the 10th of June, 1760.

Whereas, many ignorant and unskillful Persons in Physick and Surgery, in order to gain a subsistence, do take upon themselves to administer Physick, and practice Surgery in the City of New York, to the endangering of the Lives and Limbs of their Patients; and many poor and ignorant Persons inhabiting the said City, who have been persuaded to become their Patients, have been great sufferers thereby: For preventing such Abuses for the Future;

I. Be it Enacted *by his Honour the Lieutenant-Governor, the Council, and the General Assembly, and it is hereby* Enacted *by the Authority of the same,* That from and after the Publication of this Act, no Person whatsoever shall practice as a Physician or Surgeon in the said City of *New York,* before he shall first have been examined in Physick or Surgery, and approved of and admitted by one of his Majesty's Council, the Judges of the Supreme Court, the King's Attorney-General, and the Mayor of the City of *New York* for the time being, or by any three or more of them, taking to their assistance for such Examination, such proper Person or Persons as they in their discretion shall think fit. And if any candidate, after due examination of his Learning, and skill in Physick and Surgery as aforesaid, shall be approved and admitted to practice as a Physician and Surgeon, or both, the said Examiners, or any three or more of them, shall give, under their hands and Seals to the person so admitted aforesaid, a Testimonial of his Examination and Admission, and in the form following, *to wit:*

To all to whom these Presents shall come, or may concern:

KNOW YE, That we whose names are hereunto subscribed, in pursuance of an Act of the Lieutenant-Governor, and Council, and the General Assembly, made and published at *New York,* the Day of   in the year of our LORD, One Thousand Seven Hundred and   entitled, *An Act, to regulate the Practice of Physic and Surgery in the City of New York,* have duly examined   Physician (or) Surgeon, (or) Physician and Surgeon (as the case may be) and having approved of his skill, have admitted him as a Physician (or) Surgeon, (or) Physician and Surgeon to practice in the said Faculty or Faculties throughout this province of New York.

In testimony whereof, we have subscribed our Names and affixed our Seals to this Instrument, at New York, this   Day of Anno Domini, One Thousand,

II. AND BE IT FURTHER ENACTED *by the authority aforesaid,* That if any Person shall Practice in the *City of New York,* as a Physician or Surgeon, or both as Physician and Surgeon, without such testimonial as aforesaid, he shall, for every such offence forfeit the sum of Five Pounds; one-half thereof to the use of the Person or Persons who shall sue for the same, and the other Moiety to the Church Wardens and Vestrymen of the said City for the use of the Poor thereof; the said Forfeiture to be recovered with costs, before the Mayor, Recorder, or any one of the Alderman of the said City, who are hereby empowered in a summary way, to hear, try and determine any suit brought for such Forfeiture, and to give Judgment and to award Execution thereupon,

PROVIDED, That this act shall not extend to any person or persons administering Physick, or practising Surgery within the said City before the Publication hereof; or to any Person having his Majesty's Commission, and employed in his Service as a Physician or Surgeon.

[Van Schaack's Revision of Colony Laws, pp. 382-3]

(B)

AN ACT

To regulate the practice of Physic and Surgery within the colony of New Jersey.

Passed, September 26, 1772.

"WHEREAS, many ignorant and unskilful persons in physic and surgery, to gain a subsistence, do take upon themselves to administer physic, and practice surgery, in the colony of New Jersey, to the endangering of the lives and limbs of their patients; and many of his Majesty's subjects, who have been persuaded to become their patients, have been great sufferers thereby; for the prevention of such abuses for the future.

"SEC. 1. *Be it enacted by the Governor, Council, and General Assembly, and it is hereby enacted by the authority of the same,* That, from and after the publication of this act, no person whatsoever shall practice as a physician or surgeon, within this colony of New Jersey, before he shall first have been examined in physic or surgery, approved of and admitted by any two of the Judges of the Supreme Court, for the time being, taking to their assistance for such examination such proper person or persons, as they in their discretion shall think fit; for which service the said Judges of the Supreme Court as aforesaid, shall be entitled to a fee of *twenty shillings,* to be paid by the person so applying; and if any candidate, after due examination of his learning and skill in physic and surgery as aforesaid, shall be approved and admitted to practice as a physician or surgeon, or both, the said examiners, or any two, or more, shall give under their hands and seals, to the person so admitted as aforesaid, a testimonial of his examination and admission in the form following, to wit:

To all whom these presents shall come, or may concern;

KNOW YE, that we whose names are hereunto subscribed, in pursuance of an act of the Governor, Council, and General Assembly of the colony of New Jersey, made in the twelfth year of the reign of our soverign Lord King George the Third, entitled *An act to regulate the practice of physic and surgery, within the colony of New Jersey,* having duly examined   of   physician or surgeon, or physician and surgeon, to practice in the said faculty or faculties, throughout the colony of New Jersey. In testimony whereof we have hereunto subscribed our names and affixed our seals to this instrument, at   this   day of   Annoque Domini 17   .

"SEC. 2. *And be it further enacted by the authority aforesaid,* That if any person or persons shall practice as a physician or surgeon or both, within the colony of New Jersey without such testimonial as aforesaid, he shall forfeit and pay for every such offence, the sum of five pounds; one half thereof to the use of any person or persons who shall sue for the same, and the other half to the use of the poor of any city or township where such person shall so practice contrary to the tenor of this act; to be recovered in any court where sums of this amount are cognizable, with costs of suit.

"SEC. 3. Provided always, that this act shall not be construed to extend to any person or persons administering physic or practising surgery before the publication hereof, within this Colony, or to any person bearing his Majesty's commission and employed in his service as a physician or surgeon. *And provided always,* that nothing in this act shall be construed to extend to hinder any person or persons from bleeding, drawing teeth, or giving assistance to any person, for which services such persons shall not be entitled to make any charge, or recover any reward. *Provided also,* that nothing herein contained shall be construed to hinder any skilful physician or surgeon from any of the neighboring colonies being sent for upon any particular occasion, from practising on such occasion within this colony.

"SEC. 4. *And be it further enacted, by the authority aforesaid,* That any person now practising physic or surgery, or that shall hereafter be licensed as by this act is directed, shall deliver his account or bill of particulars to all and every patient in plain English words, or as nearly so as the articles will admit of; all and every of which accounts shall be liable, whenever the patient, his executors or administrators shall require, to be taxed by any one or more of the judges of the inferior court of common pleas of the county, city, or borough wherein the party complaining resides, calling to their assistance such persons therein skilled as they may think proper.

"SEC. 5. *And be it further enacted, by the authority aforesaid,* That every physician, surgeon or mountebank doctor who shall come into, and travel through this colony, and erect any stage or stages for the sale of drugs or medicines of any kind, shall for every such offence forfeit and pay the sum of twenty pounds, proclamation money; to be recovered in any court where the same may be cognizable, with costs of suit; one half to the person who will prosecute the same to effect, the other half to the use of the poor of any city, borough, ownership or precinct where the same offence shall be committed.

"SEC. 6. *And be it further enacted, by the authority aforesaid,* That this act, and every clause and article herein contained, shall continue and be in force for the space of five years, and from thence until the end of the next session of the General Assembly, and no longer."*

(C)

Although Connecticut did not pass any laws regulating the practice of physic, she was by no means unmindful of what related to the public health. The following in relation to the use of tobacco is a sample of her hygienic legislation. It is taken from the famous "Blue Laws" of 1650.

"Forasmuch as it is observed that many abuses are crept in, and committed by frequent taking of tobacko, *it is ordered by the authority of this court,* that no person under the age of twenty-one years, nor any other, that hath not already accusomed himself to the use thereof, shall take any tobacko until he hath brought a certificate under the hands of some, who are approved for knowledge and

---

* New Jersey Medical Reporter and Transactions of the New Jersey Medical Society. Edited by Joseph Parish, M.D. Vol. i. p. 282.

skill in physic, that it is useful for him, and also that he hath received a license from the court for the same. And for the regulating of those who, either by their former taking it have to theire own apprehensions made it necessary to them, or upon due advice thereof."

"*It is ordered,* That no man in this colony, after the publication hereof, shall take any tobacko, publiquely in the streets, highways, or any barn yards, or upon training days in any open places, under the penalty of six pence for each offence against this order in any of the particulars thereof, to be paid without gainsaying, upon conviction by testimony of *one* witness, that is without just exception, and before any one magistrate. And the constables in the several towns are required to make presentment to each particular court of such as they do understand and can evict to be transgressors of this order."

In another section of the laws providing for the due punishment of unprofitable waste of time, there is the following item:

"*It is ordered by this court,* and the authority thereof, That no person, householder or other, shall spend his time idly or unprofitably under paine of such punishment as this court shall think meete to inflict; and for this it is ordered that the constable of every place shall use special care and diligence, to take knowledge of offenders of this kinde, especially of common coasters, unprofitable fowlers, and *tobacko takers,* and present the same unto any magistrate." See an Essay on Tobacco, by J. Smyth Rogers, M.D. New York, 1811, p. 29.

(D)

In Henning's Statutes at Large of Virginia, vol. 4, page 509, is

AN ACT

For regulating the fees and accounts for Practicers of Physic.

Passed August, 1736.

I. WHEREAS, the practice of physic in this colony, is most commonly taken up and followed, by surgeons, apothecaries, or such as have only served apprenticeships to those trades, who often prove

very unskilful in the art of a physician; and yet do demand excessive fees, and expect unreasonable prices for the medicines which
they administer, and as too often, for the sake of making up long
and expensive bills, load their patients with greater quantities
thereof, than are necessary or useful, concealing all their compositions, as well to prevent the discovery of their practice, as of the
true value of what they administer; which is become a grievance,
dangerous and intolerable, as well to former sort of people, as others,
and doth require the most effectual remedy that the nature of the
thing will admit:

II. *Be it therefore enacted,* by the Lieutenant Governor, Council, and Burgesses, of this present General Assembly, and it is
hereby enacted, by the authority of the same, That from and after
the passing of this act, no practicer in physic, in any action or suit
whatsoever, hereafter to be commenced in any court of record in
this colony, shall recover, for visiting any sick person, more than
the rates hereafter mentioned: that is to say,

Surgeons and opothecaries, who have served an apprenticeship
to those trades, shall be allowed:

	£.	s.	d.
For every visit and prescription, in town or within five miles,	00	5	00
For every mile, above five, and under ten,	00	1	00
For every visit, of ten miles,	00	10	00
And for every mile, above ten,	00	00	06
With an allowance for all ferriages in their journeys. To surgeons, for a simple fracture, and the cure thereof,	02	00	00
For a compound fracture and the cure thereof,	04	00	00

But those persons who have studied physic in any University,
and taken any degree therein, shall be allowed,

	£.	s.	d.
For every visit, and prescription, in any town, or within five miles,	00	10	00
If above five miles, for every mile more, under ten,	00	1	00
For a visit, if not above ten miles,	1	00	00
And for every mile, above ten,	00	1	00
With an allowance of ferriages, as before.			

III. And to the end the true value of the medicines administered by any practicer in physic, may be better known, and judged of. *Be it further enacted* by the authority aforesaid, That whenever any pills, bolus, portion, draught, electuary, decoction, or any medicines, in any form whatsoever, shall be administered to any sick person, the person administering the same shall, at the same time, deliver in his bill, expressing every particular thing made up therein; or if the medicine administered, be a simple, or compound, directed in the dispensatories, the true name thereof shall be expressed in the same bill, together with the quantities and prices, in both cases. And in failure thereof, such practicer, or any apothecary, making up the prescription of another, shall be non-suited, in any action or suit hereafter commenced, which shall be grounded upon such bill or bills; nor shall any book, or account, of any practicer in physic, or any apothecary, be permitted to be given in evidence, before a court; unless the article therein contained, be charged according to the directions of this act.

IV. *And be it further enacted,* by the authority aforesaid, That this act shall continue and be in force for and during two years, next after the passing thereof, and from thence to the end of the next session of Assembly.

(E)

AN ACT

To prevent infectious Distempers in the Counties therein mentioned.

Passed 24th March, 1772.

WHEREAS, The Practice of Inoculation for the Small Pox is carried on in Houses situate near the public Roads and Landing Places in the Counties of *Westchester, Dutchess* and *Orange,* greatly prejudicial to the Inhabitants thereof:

I. BE IT THEREFORE ENACTED, by his Excellency the Governor, the Council, and the General Assembly, and it is hereby Enacted by the Authority of the same, That in case any Person or Persons whatsoever, shall carry on the Practice of Inoculation for the Small

Pox in the Counties of *Westchester* and *Dutchess,* and in the Pre-cincts of *Goshen* or *Cornwall,* in the County of *Orange,* within the Distance of a quarter of a mile of any Dwelling House, Public Road or Landing Place, within the Counties aforesaid, shall forfeit the sum of *Five Pounds* for every such offence; which offence is to be proved by two credible Witnesses before any one of his Majesty's Justices of the Peace, within the Counties aforesaid, where the of-fence is committed; who is hereby impowered to hear, try and de-termine the said offence or offences, to give judgment and grant Execution for the same with Costs of suit against the offender or offenders Goods and Chattels, within the space of three months, one-third of the said Forfeiture to be for the Prosecutor, and the other two-thirds for the use of the Poor of the Town, Borough, Manor or Precinct within the said Counties where the offence shall be committed; and in case no goods or chattels can be found, then the offender or offenders shall be committed to Goal for the space of three months, without Bail or Mainprize, except such Fine as aforesaid shall be sooner paid.

II. PROVIDED ALWAYS, *and be it further Enacted by the Authority aforesaid,* That nothing herein contained shall be construed to pre-vent any private Family from being Inoculated in their own Dwell-ing Houses within the said Counties and Precincts, provided the same shall be a quarter of a mile distant at least from any public Landing; and provided also, that no person whatsoever shall be there Inoculated, except their own Family; anything herein con-tained to the contrary notwithstanding.

This Act to continue in force until the First day of *February,* one thousand seven hundred and seventy-five.

AN ACT

For regulating the Practice of Inoculation for the Small Pox in the City of Albany.

Passed the 6th of February, 1773.

I. BE IT ENACTED, by his Excellency the Governor, the Council, and the General Assembly, and it is hereby Enacted by the Author-ity of the same, That from and after the publication of this Act, and during the continuance thereof, no person or Persons whatever, shall make use of any House or Building within the City of *Albany*, as a Hospital or House of Reception, for receiving People with Intent to inoculate or cause them to be inoculated for the Small Pox, unless by a License previously obtained from the Mayor, Recorder, Aldermen, and Commonalty of the said City, in Common Council convened: *Provided Always,* That nothing in this Act shall extend, or be construed to deprive or prevent any person or persons from inoculating any Person or Persons belonging to his, her or their family, in their own House.

II. AND BE IT FURTHER ENACTED, That if any Person or Persons shall offend contrary to the true Intent and Meaning of this Act, such offender or offenders shall be liable to and pay a Fine of *Fifty Pounds,* to be recovered in any Court of Record in the City and County of *Albany,* One Half to go to the Informer, and the other to the Poor of the City.

The publishers wish to thank Dr. Charles F. Fishback for contributing the foreword to this book. Dr. Fishback took his undergraduate study at the University of Illinois and his medical training at Northwestern University. He did postgraduate work under a fellowship at Mayo Clinic and then joined the Lovelace Clinic in Albuquerque, New Mexico. After serving in the Navy during World War II, Dr. Fishback returned to the Lovelace Clinic where he is now Senior Pediatrician.